A WEEK IN
THE
ZONE

Also by Dr. Barry Sears

The Zone

Mastering the Zone

Zone Food Blocks

Zone-Perfect Meals in Minutes

The Top 100 Zone Foods

The Soy Zone

The Omega Rx Zone

What to Eat in the Zone

Zone Meals in Seconds

A WEEK IN
THE
ZONE

Barry Sears, Ph.D.

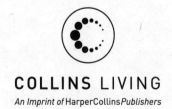

COLLINS LIVING

An Imprint of HarperCollins*Publishers*

First trade paperback edition published 2004.

Library of Congress Cataloging-in-Publication Data

Sears, Barry, 1947–
   A week in the zone / Barry Sears.—1st ed.
     p. cm.
   Includes bibliographical references and index.
   ISBN 0-06-074190-2
   1. Reducing diets. 2. Nutrition. 3. Insulin resistance. I. Title.

RM222.2.S3897 2004
613.2'5—dc22

2004041872

10 11 12 WBC/RRD 20 19 18 17 16 15 14

CONTENTS

ACKNOWLEDGMENTS

The success of the Zone books that I have written during the past five years is primarily due to my support team, which is comprised of not only my coworkers, but also my closest friends. These include my wife, Lynn Sears, who does much of the editing of my books, and my brother, Doug Sears, who has a very clear insight and understanding of how to translate cutting-edge science into easily understood terms for the general public. In addition, I wish to especially thank Deborah Kotz for her excellent advice and input in helping develop this book.

At the same time, I also have a team at ReganBooks that consistently does an outstanding job of fine-tuning my books for the general public. For this particular book, I want to give special thanks to Vanessa Stich and Cassie Jones for their excellent editing.

Of course, my greatest thanks always goes to Judith Regan, who had the courage and foresight to support the Zone, and in the process helped improve the lives of millions of people.

INTRODUCTION

Since the publication of *The Zone* 1995, more than 3 million Zone books have been sold in America. Furthermore, these books have been translated into 14 languages, making the Zone a worldwide phenomenon. The concept that hormones can be controlled by the diet is quickly becoming recognized as one of the key medical breakthroughs that will be the centerpiece for twenty-first-century health care.

Even with this growing recognition, the Zone remains misunderstood by many. Some think of the Zone as a high-protein diet, which it is not. Many more consider the Zone too difficult to follow, which it is not. What the Zone is is a powerful, yet simple to use dietary program that will allow you to lose excess body fat, reduce the likelihood of chronic disease, and enable you to live a longer and better life. All of these benefits come from your ability to use food to lower excess insulin levels.

This book represents the condensation of many of the themes that I have explored in greater detail in my previous five Zone books. It is written in such a form that makes it extraordinarily simple for you to spend a week in the Zone. Within that short time span you will experience the power of improved insulin control. That power can be yours on a lifetime basis as long as you follow the simple how-to instructions in this book.

This book answers many questions people have asked me over the past five years of how and why the Zone works. For more detailed information on various components of the Zone, I strongly refer you back to the appropriate Zone book that describes in more detail the science behind the Zone or in-depth discussions of how to cook in the Zone. At the same time, I also present here some of the newest published research that validates the Zone as your key to a better and healthier life in the new millennium. All that I ask is you try the Zone for a week. I promise you it will change your life forever.

1

WHAT IS THE ZONE?

For generations, every male on my father's side of my family suffered from a similar fate: a premature heart attack that cut their life short decades too early. After my father died in 1972 at the age of 54, I realized that I had a genetic time bomb ticking away inside me. I knew I couldn't change my genes, but I was determined to find a way to lead a normal, healthy life span.

My quest to save myself has led me to a surprisingly simple conclusion. As it turns out, the key to a longer, better life is not some magic pill or potion. It is a powerful hormone produced by your diet called insulin. My research showed that if you were able to keep insulin levels within a certain zone—not too high and not too low—you could dramatically improve your health and prevent a wide range of diseases. What's more, you could also make your body start using fat for energy, thus allowing you to lose excess body fat without feeling hungry!

So how do you begin to regulate your insulin levels and begin the journey to better health? Again, I found that the answer was simple: by eating the right combination of foods at every meal. Essentially, you need to start treating the Zone diet as a drug. Once you start taking this drug, you will automatically achieve:

- Permanent loss of excess body fat
- Dramatic reduction in the risk of chronic diseases like heart disease, diabetes, and cancer
- Improved mental and physical performance
- A longer life

The first person to recognize food as a wonder drug was Hippocrates, the father of medicine, who instructed us to "let food be your medicine, and let medicine be your food." Now some twenty-five hundred years later, we are just beginning to understand the importance of his words.

Make no mistake about it; food is a powerful drug. In fact, it may be the most powerful drug you will ever take. However, like any drug, food can help you or harm you depending on how you use it. Used correctly, food can make you more energized and healthier with the guarantee of a longer and more active life. Used incorrectly, food can become your worst enemy—robbing you of a healthy body, healthy weight, and a healthy mind, as millions of Americans are quickly finding out for themselves. Most important, if food is used improperly, it can also shorten your life.

You may think you already know how to properly use food by avoiding fat, and eating plenty of carbohydrates like pasta, bagels, bread, and rice. If you've been following these dietary guidelines, however, you may be puzzled as to why you're *gaining* rather than losing weight. Truth is, you have it backward. If you're like most Americans, you're probably eating far too many carbohydrates. This is why more than 50 percent of Americans are overweight today compared to 33 percent twenty years ago—even though we're now eating less fat than ever before. This is called the American paradox. If fat were the enemy, then we should have declared victory over obesity many years ago. The fact is that dietary fat was never the real enemy. **The real cause of our growing epidemic of obesity is excess production of the hormone insulin. It is excess insulin that makes you fat and keeps you fat.**

You are constantly reminded that a calorie is a calorie, and that weight gain is simply more calories coming in than calories going out. Since fat contains more calories per gram than does protein or carbohydrate, simple logic would dictate that removing fat from the diet should make us thinner. Such caloric thinking can be summarized as follows "if no fat touches my lips, then no fat reaches my hips." Well, it doesn't take a rocket scientist to walk on the streets of America and realize that statement simply isn't true. On the hormonal level, all calories are not created equal. The hormonal effect of a calorie of carbohydrate is different than the hormonal effect of a calorie of protein, and is still different from the hormonal effect of a calorie of fat. Each of these three nutrients has its own unique effects on your body's hormones. In the proper balance, these three nutrients are exactly what your body needs to remain healthy by keeping insulin within the Zone. When these nutrients are out of balance and insulin levels surge too high, they can wreak havoc on your body's hormonal equilibrium, resulting in weight gain, an increased likelihood of chronic disease, and acceleration of the aging process. On the other hand, if insulin levels are too low, your cells begin to starve because a certain amount of insulin is required to drive life-sustaining nutrients into your cells.

The Zone is like the story of Goldilocks and the Three Bears. One bowl of porridge was too hot (too much insulin), one bowl was too cold (too little insulin), and one was just right (the Zone).

ZONE BENEFITS

In the Zone, almost magical metabolic changes occur. Only in the Zone can you release excess fat from your fat cells to be used as fuel by your body twenty-four hours a day, allowing you to lose weight and enjoy more energy simultaneously. Only in the Zone can you reduce the likelihood of chronic disease. Only in the Zone can you live a longer life. It's as easy as eating the right combination of protein, carbohydrates, and fat at every meal and snack.

The benefits of maintaining insulin in the Zone are almost immediate, because your blood sugar is also automatically stabilized. As a result, you feel less hungry, you are more mentally alert and more energized throughout the day. Carbohydrate cravings become a thing of the past so that you can free your body from its slavery to food. How long does it take to see these benefits if you follow the basic guidelines presented in this book? No more than seven days.

With one week in the Zone, you will feel more alert, less fatigued, and never be hungry. And you will lose excess body fat at the fastest possible rate. Most important, you'll be doing everything in your power to keep yourself healthy and reduce the likelihood of developing such killers as heart disease, diabetes, and cancer. The end result is that you will live longer.

THE BASIC ZONE RULES

Although the next chapters will give you more details of the Zone program and additional tools you need to get yourself into the Zone, here is the basic starter package. To get your feet wet, read these basic Zone rules. You may even want to make a copy of this page and keep it in your wallet for reference when you're eating on the road.

Make sure every meal and snack gets you to the Zone by eating the right combination of low-fat protein, the appropriate type carbohydrate (preferably fruits and vegetables), and a little dash of "good" fat (like a sprinkling of nuts or olive oil).

1. Always eat a Zone meal within one hour after waking.
2. Try to eat five times per day: three Zone meals and two Zone snacks.
3. Never let more than five hours go by without eating a Zone meal or snack—regardless of whether you are hungry or not. In fact, the best time to eat is when you aren't hungry because that means you have stabilized your insulin levels. Afternoon and late evening snacks (which are really mini-Zone meals) are important to keep you in the Zone throughout the day.
4. Eat more fruits and vegetables (yes, these are carbohydrates) and ease off the bread, pasta, grains, and other starches. Treat breads, pasta, grains, and other starches like condiments.
5. Drink at least eight 8-ounce glasses of water every day. That's about a gallon of water.
6. If you make a mistake at a meal, don't worry about it. There's no guilt in the Zone. Just make your next meal a Zone meal to get you back where you (and your hormones) belong.

Now that wasn't so hard. In fact, you are probably telling yourself, "I can do that." If you want to jump right into the Zone, then go immediately to Chapter 5, in which you'll find a week of Zone meals for males and females. If you want a little more information about the Zone, continue to Chapter 2, and I'll show you why living in the Zone is controlled by the hormones and how those hormones are generated by the food you eat.

2

FOOD AND HORMONES: YOUR KEYS TO ENTERING THE ZONE

Entering the Zone is simply learning how to maintain the hormones generated by the food you eat within zones (not too high, not too low) from meal to meal. It's like riding a hormonal bicycle. If you can maintain your balance, you have unlimited freedom to go almost anywhere. However, if you can't balance your bicycle, you will always be falling down, never reaching your final destination—a longer and better life.

The Zone is not some mystical place or clever marketing phrase. The Zone has precise medical definitions that can be measured by simple blood tests. But the easiest test to determine whether or not you are in the Zone is to take off your clothes and take a look at yourself in front of a mirror. If you are fat and shaped like an apple, you are definitely *not* in the Zone. As you can quickly see, most Americans are not in the Zone. But even if you are thin, you can still be out of the Zone, as indicated by constant fatigue, low stamina, and persistent hunger. A quick blood test to measure your insulin levels will tell you for sure. And if they are too high, getting into the Zone will lower them.

Just because the Zone is based on treating food with the same respect that you would treat any prescription drug doesn't mean food has to taste like a drug. In fact, this book will show how incredibly easy it is to take the foods you like to eat, make a few minor adjustments, and get into the Zone on a lifetime basis.

To enter the Zone, you need to begin thinking of food in terms of three categories: protein, carbohydrates, and fats. All foods are composed of these three "macronutrients" to varying degrees: most foods contain a bulk of one group, and trace amounts of the others. Just to make sure we are talking the same language, I often tell people that "protein moves around, and carbohydrates grow in the ground." Obviously, fish and chicken are both proteins, since they move around. But what about carbohydrates? Well, pasta is a carbohydrate because it comes from wheat and that grows in the ground. What about broccoli? It grows in the ground, so it also must be a carbohydrate. And apples? They come from apple trees, which grow in the ground. That also makes an apple a carbohydrate. The fact that fruits and vegetables are carbohydrates comes as a major revelation to most Americans. One reason people are so confused about what to eat is that they often don't fully understand what they are eating.

Protein, carbohydrates, and fats all have unique hormonal impacts. Carbohydrates stimulate insulin, protein affects the hormone glucagon, and fats affect still another group of hormones called eicosanoids. How these three hormone systems impact your life is the science behind the Zone.

Let's take insulin first. Insulin is a "storage hormone." It tells the body to store incoming nutrients. Without adequate insulin, your cells starve to death and you die. On the other hand, too much insulin will make you fat, and accelerates the aging process. There are two ways to increase insulin and drive yourself out of the Zone. The first is to eat too many carbohydrates at any one meal. Carbohydrates are powerful stimulators of insulin secretion. The other is to eat too many calories at any one meal. Excess calories (especially carbohydrates) increase insulin levels because they must be stored somewhere in the body, and that demands more insulin. Furthermore, any excess calories the body cannot immediately store will be converted to fat and sent straight to your hips, stomach, or other problem areas for storage. Unfortunately, the same high levels of insulin that cause you to store fat will also block the release of any stored body fat for energy. This is why excess insulin makes you fat and keeps you fat.

On the other hand, dietary protein stimulates the release of glucagon, which has the opposite hormonal effect of insulin. Glucagon is a "mobilization hormone." It tells the body to release stored carbohydrate in the liver to replenish blood sugar levels for the brain. Without adequate levels of glucagon, you will always feel hungry and mentally fatigued because the brain is not getting enough of its primary fuel—blood sugar.

Insulin and glucagon are constantly performing this balancing act. If one hormone goes up, then the other hormone goes down. This is why the balance of protein to carbohydrate at *every* meal and snack is critical for maintaining insulin within the Zone.

Finally, there is fat. Fat has no direct effect on insulin. Nor does it have any effect on glucagon. So why not simply take all fat out of the diet? The reason is that fat has an effect on another group of hormones called eicosanoids, and these hormones also help control insulin levels. In many ways, eicosanoids are master hormones that orchestrate the functions of a vast array of other hormonal systems in your body. In a way, eicosanoids are analogous to a computer. Each of these hormones is shown below in a cartoon-like format.

The Zone is about how these three hormonal systems (insulin, glucagon, and eicosanoids) are controlled by the food you eat. The Zone is about hormonal thinking, not caloric thinking. It's a new way of looking at the food we eat, and that's what makes the Zone controversial, even though it is ultimately based on balance and moderation.

Hormones Affected by Your Diet

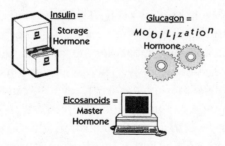

More than three million Americans have entered the Zone, and they can attest that the Zone works. More important, in the last year numerous scientific studies (see Chapter 15) by independent investigators have validated the Zone. Yet how could our government and all the nutritional "experts" have missed the boat? Because they are still thinking calorically, not hormonally.

Before you can fully understand the revolutionary implications of the Zone and all the vast benefits of being in the Zone, you need to clear your mind of many misconceptions about nutrition.

All too frequently, the dietary advice you read about in newspapers or magazines is totally conflicting, if not downright dangerous to your health. Yet the more you hear something, the more you read about it, the more you're likely to believe it. With all the news reports and TV commercials touting the wonders of bagels, pasta, and breakfast cereals, you have more than likely been piling on these fat-free carbohydrates at the expense of protein and fat. Nutritional mantras like "eat no fat," "avoid protein," and "use pasta as the main course" dance around in your head at every meal. What passes as nutritional "wisdom" can sabotage your weight and health unless you understand some Zone facts that are based on hormonal thinking. These facts upset much of this nutritional mythology that currently pervades America.

ZONE FACT #1: IT IS EXCESS INSULIN THAT MAKES YOU FAT AND KEEPS YOU FAT

You can't get fat by eating dietary fat alone—although none of us could live on only olive oil and vegetable shortening anyway. This is because dietary fat has no direct effect on insulin. So what does make you fat? It's excess levels of insulin. There are two ways to increase insulin levels in your body. The first is by eating too many fat-free carbohydrates at any one meal. The other is by eating too many calories at any one meal. In the past 15 years, Americans have done both simultaneously. This is why we have become the fattest people on the face of the earth, even though we are eating less fat than we were 15 years ago. Think of it this way: the best way to fatten cattle is to raise their insulin levels by feeding them excessive amounts of low-fat grain. By the same token, the best way to fatten humans is to raise their insulin levels by feeding them excessive amounts of low-fat grain, but now in the form of pasta and bagels.

ZONE FACT #2: YOUR STOMACH IS POLITICALLY INCORRECT

Your stomach is one giant vat of acid that can't tell one carbohydrate from another. From that perspective, one Snickers bar will be broken down by the stomach into the same amount of carbohydrate as found in 2 ounces of pasta. Now, you probably wouldn't eat four Snickers bars at one sitting, but it's very easy to eat 8 ounces of pasta. And that 8 ounces of pasta will send your insulin levels soaring. The more insulin you produce, the fatter you become.

ZONE FACT #3: EVERYONE IS NOT GENETICALLY THE SAME

Life just isn't fair. Genetically, some of us are luckier than others when it comes to handling dietary carbohydrates. For some, it seems as if just looking at a potato will make us fat. Others can eat all the potato chips they want without gaining an ounce because they don't make very much insulin when they eat carbohydrates. You know who these people are, and they probably aren't your closest friends. Unfortunately, about 75 percent of us have a relatively strong insulin response to carbohydrates, which means that our bodies make too much insulin if they overconsume carbohydrates. Excess insulin production makes our blood sugar fall too quickly, which makes us tired, fatigued, and hungry for more carbohydrates. (This is the biochemical reason that you crave carbohydrates all day long.) The amount of carbohydrates your body can handle properly without an excessive insulin response depends on your own genetic makeup. How can you tell if you're sensitive to carbohydrates? Eat a big pasta meal at noon, and then see how you feel three hours later. If you are hungry and having trouble staying awake, then you fall into the 75 percent of the population who are not so genetically lucky.

ZONE FACT #4: UNTIL 10,000 YEARS AGO, THERE WERE NO GRAINS ON EARTH

We are told that bread is the staff of life. The fact is that modern man has not changed, to any great extent, genetically for the past 100,000 years. For most of the time that humans have lived on the planet, we ate only two food groups: low-fat protein, and fruits and vegetables. The Zone is the diet that we were genetically designed to eat. Grains were simply not part of the diet that modern man evolved from. When grains were introduced 10,000 years ago, three things happened immediately:

1. Mankind shrank in size due to the lack of adequate protein.
2. Diseases of "modern civilization," such as heart attacks and arthritis, first appeared and were routinely reported in the medical textbooks of ancient Egypt.
3. Obesity became prevalent. In fact, it is estimated that the ancient Egyptians—with their grain-based diets—had about the same rate of obesity as Americans do today.

Since our genes haven't changed much in the past 100,000 years, don't expect them to change much in the next 100,000 years.

ZONE FACT #5: IT TAKES FAT TO BURN FAT

If you are thinking calorically, this statement makes no sense because fat contains calories. On the other hand, if you are thinking hormonally, this statement makes perfect sense, because fat has no effect on insulin. However, the right types of fat do play an indirect role in helping lower the insulin response to carbohydrates. First, fat slows down the entry rate of carbohydrates into the bloodstream, thereby decreasing the production of insulin. Second, fat sends a hormonal signal to the brain that says, "Stop eating," and the fewer calories you eat, the less insulin you make. Third, fat makes food taste better (just ask the French). So by taking fat (which has no effect on insulin) out of the diet and replacing it with carbohydrates (which have a strong stimulatory effect on insulin), you are virtually guaranteeing that you will become fatter. However, not all fats are created equal. The best type of fat to add back into your diet is heart-healthy monounsaturated fat, found in such foods as olive oil, avocados, almonds, and macadamia nuts, and long-chain omega-3 fats, found in fish and fish oils.

ZONE FACT #6: THE PRIMARY PREDICTOR OF HEART DISEASE IS HIGH LEVELS OF INSULIN

Heart disease is the number-one killer of both men and women in America. However, the best predictor of heart disease is not high cholesterol, not high blood pressure, but elevated levels of insulin. How can you tell if you have elevated insulin? Look in the mirror. If you're fat and shaped like an apple, you have elevated insulin. However, you can be thin and still have elevated insulin. How can you tell? Have a blood test to measure your lipid levels. If you have high triglycerides (more than 150 mg idl) and low HDL cholesterol (less than 35 mg idl), you are producing too much insulin and are at increased risk for heart disease. This is why high-carbohydrate, low-fat diets can be extremely dangerous for cardiovascular patients. They may lose weight if they're eating fewer calories, but they often experience an increase in triglycerides and a decrease in HDL cholesterol, which dramatically increases cardiac risk.

ZONE FACT #7: CARBOHYDRATES ARE DRUGS THAT CAN ACCELERATE AGING

Carbohydrates are not manna from heaven. You need some carbo-hydrates at every meal for optimal brain function, but like any drug, excess carbohydrates at a meal will have a toxic side effect: the overproduction of insulin. The primary cause of aging is due to the continued production of excess insulin and its ability to acceler-ate the development of chronic disease.

ZONE FACT #8: THE ZONE IS NOT A HIGH-PROTEIN DIET

A high-protein diet is exactly that: you are eating excessive amounts of protein, often rich in saturated fat. In the Zone, you never eat more than 3 to 4 ounces of low-fat protein at any one meal. This is exactly what virtually every nutritionist recommends. Furthermore, you are always eating more carbohydrates than pro-tein in the Zone, so it's impossible for the Zone to be considered a high-protein diet. As I explain in greater detail in Chapter 14, although high-protein diets are currently popular, they are virtually

guaranteed to fail to provide permanent weight loss. And if followed for any extended period of time, high-protein diets will most
likely increase your risk for heart disease.

WHAT THE ZONE CAN DO FOR YOU

With this quick primer on food and hormones, let's explore what
the Zone can do for you in both the short term and the long term.
If you're following the Zone, here are some of the immediate benefits you will observe during your first week. You will:

Think Better

By keeping your blood sugar levels stable throughout the day,
your brain is constantly being supplied with energy. You'll find
that you have a better ability to concentrate, and won't suffer from
that mental haziness that can occur two to three hours (if not
sooner) after eating a high-carbohydrate meal. You will feel more
refreshed in the morning and more energized throughout the day.
Afternoon slumps will be a thing of the past, as will be carbohydrate cravings.

Perform Better

By stabilizing insulin levels, you will be able to access stored
body fat as a virtually unlimited supply of energy throughout the
day. (Remember that excess insulin prevents the release of stored
body fat.)

Look Better

Don't expect a lot of immediate weight loss on the Zone during
the first week of the program, because it's physically impossible to
lose more than 1 to 1½ pounds of body fat per week. However, all
of the weight you will lose in the Zone will be pure fat, as opposed
to water and muscle. Your body composition will change, and as a
consequence, your clothes will start fitting better even though your
scale isn't moving that much.

Feel Better

You'll feel less cranky and moody in between meals because you won't experience those sugar lows that make you tired, hungry, and irritable. Overall, you'll feel like your life is on an even keel—a sign that your hormones are, too.

Experience Fewer Carbohydrate Cravings and Become Totally Satisfied with Fewer Calories

Carbohydrate cravings are not an indication that you are a weak-willed person. They are simply a consequence of making a poor hormonal choice at your last meal. Once you learn to make Zone meals, the underlying cause of carbohydrate cravings will disappear. As an added benefit of being in the Zone, you'll be eating fewer calories than you're used to, but won't feel as hungry because your blood sugar levels are stabilized. Recent studies at Harvard Medical School have confirmed this.

While these are great short-term benefits, the real reason you want to make the Zone an integral part of your life is because it can result in a vast number of long-term health benefits that come with better insulin control. These include:

1. **You will achieve permanent fat loss.** The only way to control your weight is to control your insulin levels. In the Zone, you will begin shedding all the excess body fat you need to lose: Many readers who have followed the plan have lost 20, 40, or even in some cases, more than 100 pounds. More important, they have kept those pounds off.
2. **You will reduce the risk of heart disease.** As you decrease insulin levels, your risk of heart disease plummets. This was demonstrated in a study published in the *Journal of the American Medical Association* that found that insulin levels are far more predictive for the development of heart disease than any other risk factor.
3. **You will be less likely to develop adult-onset (Type 2) diabetes.** We usually think of diabetes as a disease in which you

make no insulin. This is called Type 1 diabetes. However, more than 90 percent of all diabetics have the opposite problem: they make too much insulin. They are known as Type 2 diabetics, and now number some 15 million Americans. Clinical studies have shown that the Zone lowers excess insulin levels in Type 2 diabetics within four days.

4. **You will be protected from arthritis and osteoporosis.** Lowering insulin can alleviate tissue inflammation, because reduced insulin levels also mean reduced levels of the building blocks of pain-producing eicosanoids. By decreasing these eicosanoids, you relieve the pain and inflammation associated with arthritis. Essentially, the Zone works in much the same way as aspirin: both control pain by controlling eicosanoids. It has also been shown that increased protein consumption actually decreases the number of hip fractures in post-menopausal women.

5. **You may reduce the risk of developing breast cancer.** A number of studies have found an association between high insulin levels and the increased risk of breast cancer. This is coupled with new research from Harvard Medical School demonstrating that the more protein (and less carbohydrates) a woman consumes, the better her survival rate after breast cancer.

6. **You'll get fewer infections.** Adequate protein ensures proper functioning of the immune system, the body's natural defense mechanism against disease. Many people on high-carbohydrate diets have suppressed immune systems and are more susceptible to infection because of excess insulin levels. They're more likely to get sick (not to mention catching more colds and the flu) than people getting adequate protein throughout the day.

Bottom line, if you want to live a longer and better life, entering the Zone is your best and safest drug. But like any drug, it only works if you take the recommended dose at the right time.

3

GETTING STARTED
IN THE ZONE

Now that you understand how protein, carbohydrates, and fats work together to control your hormone levels, your body fat composition, and your overall health, you can begin making Zone-perfect meals. These meals will be your passport to the Zone.

GETTING READY TO MAKE ZONE MEALS

Ironically, the Zone is based on two terms your grandmother told you: balance and moderation. You balance your plate at every meal, and never eat too many calories at a meal. The only tools you need are the palm of your hand and your eye.

START WITH PROTEIN

Every Zone meal starts with making sure that you have an adequate serving of low-fat protein. There are several reasons for this. The first is that your body needs a constant supply of dietary protein to replace the protein that is constantly lost from your body on a daily basis. Without adequate incoming protein, your muscles weaken and your immune system becomes far less effective. Second, protein stimulates the release of glucagon. Recall that glucagon is a mobilization hormone that tells the body to release stored carbohydrates from the liver to maintain adequate blood sugar levels for the brain. Without adequate protein in a meal, hunger (due to the inability to maintain blood sugar levels) will result in two to three hours after a meal. Finally, glucagon acts as a brake on excess insulin secretion. If glucagon levels increase, then insulin levels decrease. By stimulating the release of enough glucagon with adequate levels of protein, you now have an ideal control mechanism to prevent too much insulin from being released.

Finally, you always want to use low-fat protein. Why? Because you will always be adding a dash of monounsaturated fat to a Zone meal, and using low-fat protein means you can control the composition of your fat instead of overconsuming saturated fat.

A very common misconception about the Zone is that you have to eat animal protein. That's simply not true. You do have to consume adequate protein, but for a vegetarian that is very easy to achieve eating egg whites, low-fat dairy products, tofu, or soy meat substitutes. As I will explain in Chapter 8, using soy products as your primary protein source may actually be the healthiest version of the Zone for a longer life.

The first step of Zone meal preparation is to *never* consume any more low-fat protein at a meal than you can fit on the palm of your hand. And before you get too excited, that amount also means the thickness of your hand. For most American females, this is 3 ounces of low-fat protein, and for most American males this is about 4 ounces of low-fat protein. Unless you are very active, your body can't utilize any more protein than that at a single sitting: any excess protein will be converted to fat. You always want to use low-fat protein for Zone meals to keep the amount of saturated fat to a minimum (since it can indirectly increase insulin levels). What are some good sources of low-fat protein? Many of your best choices follow.

Best Protein Choices

- Skinless chicken
- Turkey
- Fish
- Very lean cuts of meat
- Egg whites

- Low-fat dairy products
- Tofu
- Soy meat substitutes

BALANCE WITH CARBOHYDRATES

Now that you have your protein portion for your Zone meal, you must balance the protein with carbohydrates. Unfortunately, most Americans have no idea what carbohydrates actually are. Many people think of them as only pasta and sweets, whereas in reality they also include fruits and vegetables. The fact that a fruit or vegetable is also a carbohydrate is a major revelation to most Americans. However, not all carbohydrates are equal in their ability to stimulate insulin. Some are "favorable" carbohydrates that have a low capacity to stimulate insulin, and others are "favorable" carbohydrates that have a high capacity to stimulate insulin. Since the name of the game is insulin control, you want to make sure that most of your carbohydrate choices come from favorable carbohydrates (primarily fruits and vegetables), and treat unfavorable carbohydrates (such as grains and starches) like condiments.

This definition of favorable and unfavorable is based on the concept of the *glycemic load.* That is calculated from the combination of both the density of the carbohydrate in a given volume, and the rate at which it will enter the bloodstream. More details about glycemic load are found in my book *The Zone*, but for now all you need to know is that the higher the glycemic load of a given volume of carbohydrate, the greater its ability to stimulate insulin.

Vegetables (except for corn and carrots) always have a low glycemic load, whereas fruits (except for bananas and raisins) will usually have an intermediate glycemic load. Starches and grains (except for oatmeal and barley, which are very rich in soluble fiber) have very high glycemic loads. Therefore, as you balance the protein on your plate, do so with a lot of vegetables, some fruits, and just a small amount of grains and starches. Below are listed some of the favorable and unfavorable carbohydrates.

Favorable and Unfavorable Carbohydrates

Favorable (have a lower effect on insulin)
Most vegetables (except corn and carrots)
Most fruits (except bananas and raisins)
Selected grains (oatmeal and barley)

Unfavorable (have a greater effect on insulin)
Grains and starches (pasta, bread, bagels, cereals, potatoes, etc.)
Selected fruits (bananas, raisins, etc.)
Selected vegetables (corn and carrots)

As you can readily see, a good portion of your current diet is probably heavy on large amounts of unfavorable carbohydrates without adequate levels of low-fat protein. That's a surefire prescription for elevated insulin, which means you are getting fatter and less healthy with each meal.

ADD FAT

Once you have balanced your plate with low-fat protein and favorable carbohydrates, there is one more thing to add before it's truly a Zone meal—fat. Remember, it takes fat to burn fat. But like carbohydrates, all fats are not equal.

There are two types of fats that fall into the category of "good" fats. These are monounsaturated fats and long-chain omega-3 fats. You get monounsaturated fats from olive oil, selected nuts, and avocados. Long-chain omega-3 fats come from fish and fish oils (like the cod liver oil your grandmother told you to take). These are exceptionally powerful allies in your quest for a longer life, as described in greater detail in my other books. But for the moment, just think of them as good fats.

However, there are some fats you want to restrict in your diet. These are saturated fats, trans fats, and arachidonic acid. I consider these to be really "bad" fats. You find saturated fats in fatty cuts of red meat and high-fat dairy products. Another type of fat to avoid is trans fats. These artificial fats were created by the food industry and are found in virtually all processed foods. Any time you see the words "partially hydrogenated vegetable oil," you know that food contains trans fats. These alien fats make processed food more stable (why do you think your Twinkie is still good after a year in your pocket?). Furthermore, Harvard Medical School has shown that the more trans fats you eat, the more at risk you are for heart disease. Finally, there is arachidonic acid, which is found primarily in fatty red meats, egg yolks, and organ meats. This particular polyunsaturated fat may be the most dangerous fat known when consumed in excess. In fact, you can inject virtually every type of fat (even saturated fat and cholesterol) into rabbits, and nothing happens. However, if you inject arachidonic acid into the same rabbits, they are dead within three minutes. The human body needs some arachidonic acid, but too much can be toxic. Ironically, the higher your insulin levels, the more your body is stimulated to make increased levels of arachidonic acid.

Listed below are both the "good" and "bad" fats for the Zone.

"GOOD" AND "BAD" FATS

Good Fats (monounsaturated fats and long-chain omega-3 fats)
Olive oil
Almonds
Avocados
Fish oils

Bad fats (saturated fats, trans fats, and arachidonic acid)
Fatty red meat
Egg yolks
Organ meats
Processed foods (rich in trans fats)

LET'S GET STARTED

Now that you have an idea of what types of protein, carbohydrate, and fat you will be using to make Zone meals, let me show you how easy it really is.

First, take your plate and divide it into three sections. On one-third of the plate put some low-fat protein that is no bigger or thicker than the palm of your hand. Then fill the other two-thirds of the plate until it is overflowing with fruits and vegetables. Then add a dash (that's a small amount) of monounsaturated fat, like olive oil, slivered almonds, or even guacamole. There you have it: a Zone meal.

I hope you can see that putting together a Zone meal isn't rocket science. But the key is consistency, since the hormonal benefits of each meal will only last four to six hours. You have to eat, so you might as well get the best hormonal bang for the buck out of each meal.

This means always balancing protein and carbohydrate at every meal and snack. For example, you can't have all of your protein in one meal and all of your carbohydrate in the next meal, because your insulin levels will swing all over the place. Consider your food like a medication. You have to take the right dose at the right time. Would you take a week's worth of drugs on Saturday afternoon? Of course not. And if you are taking your drug every day, would you take 5 mg in the morning, 500 mg at noon, and 28 mg in the evening? Of course not. You would try the best you could to take the same amount of the drug each time. Why? You want to keep the drug within a Zone; not too high (where it's toxic), nor too low (where it doesn't work). Treat food the same way. Your goal is to maintain insulin in a similar Zone by balancing protein and carbohydrate and using only your eye and the palm of your hand to do it.

A DAY IN THE ZONE

So now that we know the basic rules, let's see what a typical day in the Zone for a typical American female might look like, using the Zone rules discussed in Chapter 1:

Breakfast

A 6-egg-white omelet mixed with some asparagus and 2 teaspoons of olive oil. The breakfast would also include ⅔ cup of slow-cooked oatmeal and a cup of strawberries.

Lunch

A grilled chicken salad with 3 ounces of chicken breast, some olive oil and vinegar dressing, and fresh fruit for dessert.

Late-afternoon snack

2 hard-boiled eggs in which the yolks have been removed and replaced with hummus (mashed chickpeas and olive oil).

Dinner

5 ounces of salmon covered with a tablespoon of slivered almonds, two cups of steamed vegetables, and a cup of mixed berries for dessert.

Late-night snack

1 ounce of soft cheese and a glass of wine (or a small piece of fruit if you don't drink).

The first thing you notice is that this is real food. The second thing is that it's also a lot of food, which means you'll never be hungry. The third thing is that it's exceptionally rich in vegetables and fruits. And the final thing, which is not so obvious, is that the total calorie content for your day in the Zone is about 1,200 calories. This is what I call the Zone paradox. **You'll eat a lot of food without hunger, fatigue, or deprivation and without consuming a lot of calories.** Most important, if you eat all the food, you are greatly increasing your chance for a longer life by keeping your overall calorie count at the level consistent with maximum longevity (see Chapter 8 for more details). Keep in mind that the typical American male would eat similar foods, only each meal should be 25 percent larger to supply the 1,500 calories he would need on a daily basis.

ZONE MEAL TIMING

Meal timing is critically important for staying in the Zone, just like taking a drug. Following the Zone, you try to eat five times per day (three meals and two snacks). Plan your day accordingly, just like you schedule appointments, so you never let more than five waking hours go by without eating a Zone meal or snack. A typical meal schedule might be as follows: if you wake up at 6:00, then eat a Zone breakfast by 7:00 (as you will see from the recipes in this book, this is a big breakfast). Five hours later, it's noon, and time for lunch, which will be another big meal. Most people won't eat dinner before 7:00, which is more than five hours after lunch, so have a snack in the late afternoon. After eating your dinner at 7:00, make sure you have one final late-night snack before you go to bed, because your brain stills needs blood sugar during your eight hours of sleep. That's a typical day in the Zone.

TIMING OF ZONE MEALS

Meal	Timing	Approximate Time
Breakfast	Within 1 hour after waking	7:00 A.M.
Lunch	Within 5 hours after breakfast	12:00 P.M.
Late-afternoon snack	Within 5 hours after lunch	5:00 P.M.
Dinner	Within 2–3 hours after snack	7:00 P.M.
Late-night snack	Before bed	11:00 P.M.

Following this program, at the end of a day in the Zone you have consumed adequate amounts of high-quality protein, extraordinary levels of vitamins and minerals from vegetables and fruits, and the same absolute amount of fat usually consumed in most vegetarian diets. You weren't hungry or fatigued because you controlled blood sugar and thus the brain was constantly supplied with the only fuel source (blood glucose) it can use. Furthermore, you didn't feel deprived because each of the meals contained large volumes of food. In fact, the size of each Zone meal can be very intimidating, because when you replace grains and starches with carbohydrates such as fruits and vegetables, the carbohydrate volumes on your plate quickly increase in size.

THE BATTLE OF THE FOOD PYRAMIDS

Now that you know what Zone meals look like, we can put this into graphic form by constructing the Zone Food Pyramid, as shown below.

As you can quickly see, using the Zone Food Pyramid, you are consuming a lot of vegetables and fruits. In fact, you would be consuming about 10 to 15 servings per day. The U.S. government recommends three to five servings per day, and virtually no one in America eats that amount. The next level in the Zone Food Pyramid is adequate amounts of low-fat protein. Notice I didn't say animal protein, because low-fat protein can also include tofu, soy protein meat substitutes, and isolated protein powder. Further up the Zone Food Pyramid is the addition of monounsaturated fats. Finally, at the top of the Zone Food Pyramid, are grains and starches, used only

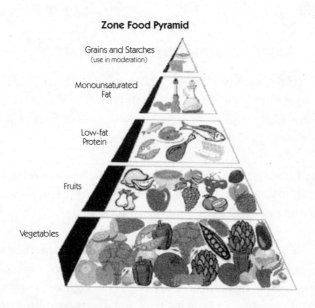

Zone Food Pyramid

Grains and Starches
(use in moderation)

Monounsaturated
Fat

Low-fat
Protein

Fruits

Vegetables

in moderation. As you can see, nothing is ever forbidden in the Zone; you just have to eat unfavorable foods in moderation.

So now we can compare the Zone Food Pyramid with the USDA Food Pyramid.

Comparison of the Food Pyramids

When you look at carbohydrates from the Zone Pyramid perspective, it becomes very clear why the USDA Food Pyramid is virtually guaranteed to increase insulin levels. The government recommends eating 6 to 11 servings each day of unfavorable carbohydrates, such as grains and starches. Using the Zone Food Pyramid, you might consume 2 servings. The government also recommends a minimum of 3 to 5 small servings of fruits and vegetables per day. Following the Zone Food Pyramid, you would eat 10 to 15 servings per day. Even though you are eating more *servings* of carbohydrates in the Zone, you are reducing your total *carbohydrate intake* by about 50 percent at the same time, because of the lower carbohydrate content of vegetables and fruits. This 50 percent reduction in carbohydrate consumption also represents a 50 percent reduction of insulin secretion, with a corresponding increase in your chances of living a longer and healthier life at your ideal body weight.

WHY GRANDMOTHER WAS RIGHT

Now that I have gone into how to eat in the Zone in more detail, you begin to understand that your grandmother's dietary advice was based on hormonal thinking. Remember the four nutritional pearls of wisdom she told you.

1. **Eat small meals throughout the day.** One of the best ways to maintain insulin levels in the Zone is not to eat too much carbohydrate or protein at any one meal. Although carbohydrate has a strong effect on insulin release, protein is also a weak stimulator of its release (however, protein has a strong impact on the release of glucagon, which inhibits insulin). By not overconsuming either protein or carbohydrate, you are well on your way to better insulin control as long as your meal is moderate in size.

2. **Have some protein at every meal.** The primary hormonal role of protein is to stimulate the release of glucagon, which mobilizes the release of stored carbohydrates so that your brain can use them for energy. In addition, glucagon also reduces the output of insulin. Using the palm of your hand (and its thickness) is a good indicator of the maximum amount of protein you should consume at any meal.

3. **Always eat your vegetables and fruits.** Now you know these carbohydrates will have a lower impact on insulin release because these are more favorable carbohydrates with a decreased glycemic load compared to grains and starches. This is also good common sense, since most of your vitamins and minerals come from vegetables and fruits. By eating primarily vegetables and fruits, you're automatically controlling the amount of carbohydrates you eat at any given meal. What's more, the fiber in these low-density carbohydrates slows digestion and lowers the rate of insulin secretion.

4. **Take your cod liver oil.** I know nothing is higher on the "yecch" scale than cod liver oil. However, it does contain long-chain omega-3 fatty acids that do a great job of keeping insulin under control and are critically important for your cardiovascular and immune function. Furthermore, they are also critically important for your brain (that's why they call fish and fish oil "brain food"). You can still hold your nose and take your cod liver oil like your grandmother did, or you can opt for a more palatable choice in the form of salmon, which is rich in the same fatty acids, or a new generation of almost tasteless fish oils.

I hope you now realize that your grandmother was actually describing how to reach the Zone. In fact, she was at the cutting edge of twenty-first-century biotechnology when it came to insulin control.

At this point, you are probably again saying that magical phrase, "I can do that." All you have to do is use the palm of your hand and be able to tell time. If you can, then living in the Zone on a lifetime basis is going to be incredibly easy.

4

A ZONE MAKEOVER FOR YOUR KITCHEN

You're about to start your week in the Zone, but first you need the proper preparation. That's what this chapter is all about: readying your kitchen to become a food pharmacy.

During the first week that you're in the Zone, you should try to make your kitchen as Zone-friendly as possible. That means taking certain "Zone-hostile" foods out of your pantry, refrigerator, and freezer and replacing them with foods that fit into your new Zone eating plan.

This way, every time you open the refrigerator door you'll be pulling out a drug as powerful as any that your doctor can prescribe. You'll be using these Zone-friendly foods to lose weight and ward off illness. You'll get a powerful burst of energy from better insulin control that will keep you mentally and physically alert throughout the day. Follow these simple steps and you'll be on your way to a lifetime of better health.

Note: These rules apply to the first week that you're in the Zone. I'm trying to make your first experience with the Zone easier by taking away all foods that are considered high-density carbohydrates—meaning they have a lot of carbohydrates packed into a small amount of space. You don't need to banish Zone-hostile foods forever. After the first week, you can add them back in small amounts and still stay in the Zone.

THE BIG CLEAR-AWAY

The first thing you want to do is temporarily remove all the potentially dangerous foods from your kitchen that will drive you out of the Zone. Take all unfavorable carbohydrates like pasta, rice, dry cereal, pancake and cookie mixes, breads, and bagels and put them in a bag. I'd also like you to do the same with any dried fruit you might have, since these also are concentrated sources of carbohydrates. Then store them in a taped box in a dark corner of your basement where you aren't likely to venture in the next week. Do the same for any breadmakers, pasta machines, and juicers you own.

MAKE A FAT SWITCH

Get rid of vegetable oil, vegetable shortening, butter, whole-milk dairy products, and any other foods that contain high amounts of saturated and omega-6 polyunsaturated fats. Replace the vegetable oils and shortenings with olive oil and nut butters (almond is the best) that are rich in monounsaturated fat. Replace the whole-milk dairy products with low-fat cottage cheese, low-fat milk, and part-skim ricotta cheese. Replace bologna and bacon with low-fat sources of protein like chicken, turkey, and fish. Also, stock up on soybean-based food products like meatless ground beef, soy hamburgers, and soy sausages. The key is to use low-fat protein sources so you can add back the small amounts of monounsaturated fat.

BE PICKY ABOUT PRODUCE

Even when it comes to fruits and vegetables, you need to be selective. Certain fruits and vegetables are high-density carbohydrates, which means they can raise your insulin levels as much as a cookie or candy bar. Again, I'd like you to get rid of all fruit juices and dried fruit, since they are concentrated sources of sugar. I'd also like you to avoid these Zone-hostile fruits: bananas, cranberries, dates, figs, guavas, kumquats, mangos, papayas, dried prunes, and raisins. The best choices for fruit include apples, apricots, pears, oranges, raspberries, plums, blueberries, strawberries, grapes, and grapefruit. Starchy vegetables are the most Zone-hostile and include acorn squash, beets, butternut squash, carrots, corn, French fries, parsnips, peas, and potatoes. The best choices for vegetables include dark green leafy vegetables, tomatoes, celery, mushrooms, and peppers. For a complete list, see Appendixes B and C for Zone Food Choices.

If the thought of cutting up fresh vegetables several times a day sounds too time-consuming, then stock up on frozen vegetables or purchase pre-cut vegetables. Frozen fruits and vegetables are picked when at their ripest and then quick-frozen—often within hours after harvesting. The end result is that frozen produce often has a higher vitamin content than fresh fruits and vegetables, which can sit around at distribution centers and supermarkets for days or weeks before you actually buy them. The longer fresh produce sits around, the more nutrition (especially vitamins) is lost. If you don't mind the taste of frozen produce, by all means, stock it in your freezer. Canned produce, on the other hand, will have fewer vitamins and minerals than fresh or frozen produce because it is more processed and loaded with preservatives. It's okay in a pinch if you haven't had time to get to the supermarket.

RESTOCK YOUR KITCHEN WITH ZONE STAPLES

Keeping certain staples around the house will make Zone cooking and snacking incredibly easy. Since Zone staples have a long shelf life, measured in months, you won't have to buy these as often. Slow-cooking oatmeal is one staple you should definitely have on hand, since it's one of the few grains I readily recommend on the Zone. Why is oatmeal so Zone-friendly? It's rich in soluble fiber that slows down the absorption of carbohydrate and contains an essential fatty acid that is found in mother's breast milk. The best kinds of oatmeal are called Scottish oats or Irish oatmeal, made from thick, coarse oats that take about 30 minutes to cook. The next best choice is old-fashioned oats, which take about five minutes to cook and still retain their chewy texture. (Avoid instant oatmeal, since it is more processed to make it cook faster and thus enters your bloodstream quickly, causing an insulin surge.)

One protein source that can be considered a Zone staple because of its very long shelf life is isolated protein powder. Protein powder can be added to fresh fruit shakes or vegetable soups and stews to fortify them with protein to turn them into Zone meals. Hormonally speaking, the best type of protein powder is soybean isolate, since it has the least effect on insulin and the greatest effect on glucagon. Unfortunately, this type of protein powder doesn't taste as good as other isolated protein sources such as whey, milk, or egg proteins. My suggestion is to use various combinations with the maximum amount of soy protein until you find a balance that meets your taste requirements.

Another vital Zone staple is nuts. Thousands of years ago, people ate nuts for fat before they were able to extract oil from olives and seeds. I prefer that you choose nuts that are rich in monounsaturated fats, like macadamia nuts, almonds, cashews, and pistachios. Peanuts are a good source of monounsaturated fat—though not as good as other kinds of nuts. Remember, nuts, including peanut butter, are primarily a source of fat. And you only need to eat a relatively small amount of nuts or nut butter to get a good dose of the monounsaturated fat that your body needs.

When you're stocking up on staples, don't leave out the spices. Spices make food taste better, and the more you use, the greater the taste sensation. Spices have no effect on insulin, so feel free to indulge your taste buds.

SHOPPING LIST FOR YOUR WEEK IN THE ZONE

Now it's time to take a trip to the supermarket. During your week in the Zone, you'll probably need to go shopping two or three times to ensure that you have the freshest fruits, vegetables, and protein. For instance, you can only keep fresh fish, chicken, and meat for two or three days at most in your refrigerator before they spoil, although you can freeze and rethaw them.

As you find yourself perusing through aisles of gleaming apples and stacked broccoli bunches, you'll probably notice that you're spending most of your time on the periphery of the supermarket, rather than in the inner aisles. This is no accident. The periphery usually contains fresh and frozen produce and perishable items like milk, cheese, poultry and fish, while the inner aisles contain processed foods like breakfast cereal, pasta, flour, and snack products. A good rule of thumb to follow whenever you're supermarket shopping is to spend most of your time on the periphery of the supermarket and very little time in the aisles that hold the greatest temptations. (Remember, if you don't buy it, you won't have any Zone no-no's beckoning you in the kitchen.)

The following shopping list for your week in the Zone is divided into two parts, which means you'll need to go shopping at the beginning of the week and then again in the middle of the week. The list is divided into categories to help you stay organized while you shop and to help you avoid forgetting any items.

SHOPPING LIST #1: FOR DAYS 1, 2, 3, 4

✔ Meat/Fish/Poultry

Turkey breast slices (deli-style)
Ham (deli-style)
Skinless chicken breast
Lean Canadian bacon (or turkey bacon strips or soy sausage
   links)
Tuna (canned albacore packed in water)
Flounder fillet
Lean ground beef (or ground turkey or soy burger patty)
Lean ground lamb

✔ Vegetable Protein

Soy protein powder
Tofu (firm)

✔ Fruits

Strawberries
Blueberries
Oranges

Apples
Seedless grapes
Cantaloupe
Reduced-sugar canned pineapple
Reduced-sugar canned mandarin oranges
Kiwi

✔ Vegetables

Green-leaf lettuce
Mushrooms (white, brown, or button)
Tomatoes
Broccoli florets
Yellow onions
Celery
Lettuce leaves
Green beans
Green peppers
Scallions
Red onions

✔ Beans and Legumes

Canned chickpeas
Snow peas

✔ Dairy Products

Cottage cheese
Swiss cheese
Low-fat yogurt
Parmesan cheese
Reduced-fat American cheese
Reduced-fat smoked mozzarella
Egg whites (or egg substitute)
Low-fat milk (1%)

✔ Grains

Hamburger rolls
Cooked brown rice

✔ Spices

Cinnamon
Fresh ginger
Fresh garlic
Black pepper
Lemon juice
Dried basil
Dried oregano
Cilantro
Cumin
Coriander
Celery salt

✔ Miscellaneous

Macadamia nuts
Almonds (slivered)
Olive oil
Red-wine vinegar
Cider vinegar
Soy sauce
Vegetable spray
Light mayonnaise
Dill pickles
Applesauce
Dry onion soup mix

SHOPPING LIST #2: FOR DAYS 5, 6, 7

✔ Meat/Fish/Poultry

Lean Canadian bacon (or turkey bacon strips or soy sausage links)
Lean ground beef (or substitute ground turkey or vegetable protein crumbles)
Shrimp
Skinless chicken breast
Salmon steak
Turkey bacon (or lean Canadian bacon or soy sausage links)
Tuna (canned albacore packed in water)

✔ Fruits

Unsweetened applesauce
Peaches
Oranges
Pears
Lemons
Apples
Mandarin oranges
Nectarines

✔ Vegetables

Yellow onions
Asparagus spears
Red peppers
Green peppers
Green-leaf or romaine lettuce
Broccoli florets
Tomatoes
Zucchini
Button mushrooms
Celery
Onions
Green beans

✔ Beans and Legumes

Canned kidney beans
Canned black beans
Canned chickpeas

✔ Dairy Products

Cottage cheese
Low-fat Monterey Jack cheese
Egg whites (or egg substitute)
Low-fat milk (1%)
Mozzarella cheese (shredded)

✔ Grains

Slow-cooked (steel-cut) oatmeal

✔ Spices

Nutmeg
Cinnamon
Chili powder
Garlic powder
Black pepper
Fresh garlic
Lemon juice
Dried rosemary
Dried tarragon
Dried dill
Dried chives
Dried parsley
Dried basil

✔ Miscellaneous

Almonds
Applesauce

Olive oil
Wine vinegar
Salsa or canned stewed tomatoes
Tomato sauce
Dry white wine
Vegetable spray
Light mayonnaise
Cider vinegar

Once you've completed your shopping trip, you can move on to the simple Zone meals outlined in Chapter 5. These meals, given separately for both males and females, will take you through your first seven days in the Zone. Take these "drugs" as directed, and you begin to change your life forever. They are designed to be simple and straightforward, with few ingredients and limited preparation and cooking time. Keep in mind that Chapter 5 is a very specific map that will guide you through your first week. Once you complete this week, you will find more Zone recipes in Chapter 6 and a sampling of some of the vegetarian meals from the Soy Zone in Chapter 8 that you can mix and match for all your meals and snacks for a lifetime in the Zone. Happy cooking, and Zone appetit!

5

RECIPES FOR A WEEK IN THE ZONE

Now that your kitchen is prepared and you understand the boundaries of the Zone, I want to show you what a typical week in the Zone looks like for both males and females. Each of these meals has the right balance of protein, carbohydrate, and fat, which means that each of these meals can be used like a drug to keep insulin within the Zone for the next four to six hours. More important, they're delicious, and quick and easy to prepare.

If you follow the simple (and great-tasting) meal planner outlined in the following pages, you'll have a surefire path straight into the Zone. Within one week, you'll be looking better, feeling better, and starting your body on a lifelong journey to optimum health.

TYPICAL FEMALE
Day 1

Breakfast: Fruit Salad

Ingredients
> ¾ cup low-fat cottage cheese
> 1 cup fresh or reduced-sugar canned pineapple, cubed
> ⅓ cup reduced-sugar canned mandarin oranges, drained
> 3 macadamia nuts, crushed

Instructions: Place cottage cheese in a bowl. Fold in pineapple, oranges, and nuts.

Lunch: Chef's Salad

Ingredients
1 cup green-leaf lettuce (substitute lettuce of your choice), washed, dried, and torn into large pieces
¼ cup canned chickpeas, drained and rinsed
½ cup button mushrooms, washed, dried, and coarsely chopped
½ cup celery, washed, dried, and coarsely chopped
1 tablespoon olive oil-and-vinegar dressing*
1½ ounces deli-style turkey breast, cut into strips
1½ ounces deli-style ham, cut into strips
1 ounce reduced-fat Swiss cheese (substitute any reduced-fat cheese), julienned

For Dessert
1 medium apple

Instructions: Toss lettuce with chickpeas, mushrooms, and celery. Dress, toss, and add meat and cheese. Serve apple for dessert.

*Zone oil-and-vinegar dressing contains 1 teaspoon olive oil and 2 teaspoons vinegar. Extra vinegar may be added to taste.

Dinner: Ginger Chicken

Ingredients
1 teaspoon olive oil
3 ounces boneless, skinless chicken breast, cut lengthwise into thin strips
2 cups broccoli florets, washed
1½ cups snow peas, washed
¾ cup yellow onion, peeled and chopped
1 teaspoon fresh ginger, grated

For Dessert
½ cup seedless grapes

Instructions: In a wok or large nonstick pan, heat oil over medium high heat. Add chicken and sauté, turning frequently, until lightly browned, about 5 minutes. Add broccoli, snow peas, onion, ginger, and ¼ cup water. Continue cooking, stirring often, until the chicken is done, water is reduced to a glaze, and vegetables are tender, about 20 minutes. If the pan dries out during cooking, add water in tablespoon increments to keep moist. Serve grapes for dessert.

Day 2

Breakfast: Yogurt and Fruit

Ingredients

1 ounce lean Canadian bacon (substitute 3 turkey bacon strips or 2 soy sausage links)
½ cup fresh blueberries, rinsed and drained
1 tablespoon slivered almonds
1 cup plain low-fat yogurt

Instructions: Prepare bacon or soy patties, following package instructions. Stir fruit and nuts into yogurt, and serve with bacon or links on the side.

Lunch: Tuna Salad

Ingredients

3 ounces albacore tuna packed in water, drained
¼ cup celery, washed, dried, and coarsely chopped
1 tablespoon olive oil-and-vinegar dressing*
1 or 2 lettuce leaves, washed and dried
½ cantaloupe, seeds scooped out
½ cup blueberries, rinsed and drained

Instructions: Mix tuna with celery and stir in dressing. Prepare a bed of the lettuce leaves and top with tuna mixture. Stuff cantaloupe with berries and serve for dessert.

Zone oil-and-vinegar dressing contains 1 teaspoon olive oil and 2 teaspoons vinegar. Extra vinegar may be added to taste.

Dinner: Foiled Flounder with Green Beans

Ingredients
vegetable spray
4½ ounces boneless flounder fillet (substitute mild, flaky fish of
    your choice)
2 tablespoons yellow onion, peeled and chopped
sprinkling of Parmesan cheese
¼ teaspoon freshly ground pepper, or to taste
squirt lemon juice
1½ cups fresh green beans, washed, ends removed, and halved
1 tablespoon almonds, slivered

For Dessert
1 cup fresh or reduced-sugar canned pineapple

Instructions: Preheat oven to 425°. Tear off an 18-by-12-inch piece of foil. Spray the center lightly with vegetable spray, and place fish in the center of the foil. Top with onion and sprinkle with cheese, pepper, and lemon juice. Fold foil loosely over fish, leaving ample space for air. Carefully turn up and seal the ends and the middle so that juices won't leak out. Bake in the preheated oven 18 minutes. Meanwhile, steam the green beans: in a large pot fitted with a steaming basket, bring 1 inch water to boil. Add beans to the basket and steam until crisp-tender, 10 minutes. Drain, place in serving bowl, and fold in almonds. When fish is done, carefully open foil to prevent steam burns, and remove to a plate. Serve with green beans. Serve pineapple for dessert.

Day 3

Breakfast: Fruit Smoothie

Ingredients
20 grams protein powder
1 cup blueberries
1 cup strawberries

3 macadamia nuts
4 ice cubes

Instructions: Place all ingredients in a blender and blend at high speed until smooth, about 1 minute. Add a little water if smoothie is too thick. If you prefer, eat the nuts on the side.

Lunch: Cheeseburger

Ingredients
3 ounces lean (less than 10% fat) ground beef (substitute 3 ounces ground turkey or 1 soy burger patty)
1 ounce reduced-fat American cheese (substitute cheese of choice)
1 tablespoon light mayonnaise
½ hamburger roll
1 thick tomato slice, optional
1 large lettuce leaf, optional
1 dill pickle wedge, optional

For Dessert
⅔ cup unsweetened applesauce
sprinkling of cinnamon

Instructions: Preheat broiler. Place burger on foil or rack and broil 5 minutes. Flip and continue cooking another 5 minutes for medium rare. One minute before expected doneness, top with cheese, and remove when melted. Spread mayonnaise on the roll. Top with burger, tomato, and lettuce. Serve pickle on the side. Sprinkle applesauce with cinnamon and serve for dessert.

Dinner: Vegetarian Stir-fry

Ingredients
1 teaspoon olive oil
⅔ cup vegetable protein crumbles* (substitute 4 ounces firm tofu)
1½ cups yellow onions, peeled and chopped
2 cups broccoli florets, washed

2 cups button mushrooms, washed, dried, and thinly sliced
1 ounce reduced-fat Swiss cheese, shredded

For Dessert
½ cup grapes

Instructions: Heat oil in a nonstick sauté pan or wok over medium-high heat. If using tofu, remove from wrapping, drain, and crumble. Add tofu or soy crumbles and stir until mixed with the oil. Add onions, broccoli, and mushrooms. Reduce heat to medium and stir-fry, stirring often, until vegetables are tender, about 15 minutes. Stir in cheese and heat until melted, about 1 minute. Serve grapes for dessert.

*Morningstar Farms makes Burger-Style Recipe Crumbles, which looks like ground beef and is a good vegetarian source of protein.

Day 4

Breakfast: Scrambled Eggs and Bacon

Ingredients
vegetable spray
4 egg whites (or ½ cup egg substitute)
1 teaspoon olive oil
1 tablespoon low-fat milk (optional)
1 ounce lean Canadian bacon (substitute 3 turkey bacon strips
    or 2 soy sausage links)

For Dessert
1 cup grapes
⅓ cup mandarin oranges

Instructions: Lightly coat a large nonstick pan with vegetable spray, and heat over medium flame. Beat egg whites with olive oil and milk, if desired. Pour into pan and cook, stirring often, until scrambled and fully set. Prepare bacon or soy links, following package instructions. Mix grapes and oranges and serve for dessert.

Lunch: Tofu Dip and Veggies

Ingredients
4 ounces firm tofu
1 ounce reduced-fat Swiss cheese, grated
¼ cup canned chickpeas, drained and rinsed
1 teaspoon olive oil
2 tablespoons fresh lemon juice
2 tablespoons Lipton's dry onion soup mix (substitute spices of
    your choice, to taste*)
1 medium green pepper, washed, cored, seeded, and cut in
    wedges
2 cups broccoli florets

For Dessert
Kiwi

Instructions: Drain tofu. Put tofu, cheese, chickpeas, olive oil, lemon juice, and onion soup mix in a blender. Blend until smooth. (For best flavor, refrigerate the dip at least 2 hours or overnight.) Place dip in a bowl in the center of a large plate. Arrange pepper strips and broccoli around bowl for dipping. Serve kiwi for dessert.

If you don't want to use the packaged soup mix, experiment with minced onions, garlic, or vegetable bouillon granules.

Dinner: Spiced Lamb with Vegetables

Ingredients
4½ ounces lean ground lamb
1 teaspoon cider vinegar
1 teaspoon olive oil
½ cup scallions, finely chopped
¾ cup red onions, cut in chunks
2 cups mushrooms
1½ cups tomatoes, diced
½ cup green beans, diced
1 tablespoon cilantro

2 teaspoons fresh ginger, minced
¼ teaspoon cumin
¼ teaspoon coriander
⅛ teaspoon black pepper
½ teaspoon celery salt
⅛ teaspoon cinnamon

Instructions: In a small glass bowl, combine lamb, vinegar, and spices. Cover and refrigerate for 30 minutes. Heat the oil in a medium nonstick sauté pan. Add meat mixture and vegetables. Cook, breaking meat up as it cooks, until lamb is cooked through and vegetables are tender. Spoon onto plate and serve.

Day 5

Breakfast: Old-fashioned Oatmeal

Ingredients

⅔ cup slow-cooking (steel-cut) oatmeal*
2 ounces lean Canadian bacon (substitute 6 turkey bacon strips or 2 soy sausage links)
⅓ cup unsweetened applesauce
1 tablespoon almonds, slivered
sprinkling of nutmeg
sprinkling of cinnamon
¼ cup low-fat cottage cheese

Instructions: Bring 3 cups water to a brisk boil over high heat. Add oatmeal, stirring well. When smooth and beginning to thicken, reduce heat to low and simmer for 30 minutes, stirring occasionally. While oatmeal is cooking, prepare bacon or soy patties, following package instructions. Remove oatmeal from the heat. Stir in applesauce and almonds. Sprinkle with cinnamon and nutmeg. Serve bacon and cottage cheese on the side.

*By slow cooking, we mean slow *cooking. Oatmeal that calls itself slow-cooking but takes only 5 minutes isn't the real McCoy (or per-*

haps we should say the real McCann's, a popular brand). To shorten the morning cooking time, make a big batch during the weekend, freeze, and microwave the correct amount in the morning. You may also put the oatmeal in a wide-mouth thermos with 1⅓ cups boiling water, and let it cook overnight.

Lunch: Chili (Meat or Vegetarian)

Ingredients

1 teaspoon olive oil
4½ ounces lean (less than 10%) ground beef (substitute ground turkey or 1 cup vegetable protein crumbles*)
¼ cup yellow onions, peeled and minced
1 teaspoon chili powder, or to taste
½ teaspoon garlic powder, or to taste
½ teaspoon freshly ground pepper, or to taste
1 cup salsa or stewed tomatoes with liquid
¼ cup kidney beans, drained and rinsed
Sprinkling of low-fat Monterey Jack cheese (optional)

Instructions: In a large nonstick sauté pan, heat oil over medium-high flame. Add meat and sauté, stirring often, until lightly browned, about 5 minutes. If using protein crumbles, heat until blended with oil, about 2 minutes. Add onions, chili powder, garlic powder, pepper, salsa, and kidney beans. Simmer, stirring occasionally, until onion is wilted and flavors are blended, about 20 minutes. Place in bowl and top with cheese, if desired.

*Morningstar Farms makes Burger Style Recipe Crumbles, which look like ground beef and are a good vegetarian source of protein.

Dinner: Shrimp Scampi with Vegetables

Ingredients

1 teaspoon olive oil
1 cup asparagus spears, washed, woody bases discarded, and bias-sliced into 1-inch-long pieces
¾ cup yellow onions, peeled and finely chopped

1 medium green pepper, washed, cored, seeded, and roughly
    chopped
2 cloves garlic, peeled and minced, or to taste
4½ ounces shrimp, shelled and deveined
¼ cup dry white wine (optional)
1–2 teaspoons lemon juice, or to taste
2 lemon wedges, optional

For Dessert
1 medium peach

Instructions: In a large nonstick pan, heat oil over medium-high heat. Sauté asparagus, onions, green pepper, and garlic, stirring often until tender, about 10 minutes. Add shrimp, white wine, and lemon juice. Lower heat to medium and cook 5 minutes, stirring often, until shrimp are pink. Place on plate and garnish with lemon wedges. Serve peach for dessert.

Day 6

Breakfast: Spanish Omelet

Ingredients
vegetable spray
2 tablespoons yellow onion, peeled and finely chopped*
2 tablespoons green pepper, cored, seeded, and roughly
    chopped*
4 large egg whites (or ½ cup egg substitute)
1 tablespoon low-fat milk (optional)
1 teaspoon chili powder, or to taste (optional)
1 teaspoon olive oil
¼ cup canned black beans, drained
1 ounce low-fat Monterey Jack cheese, shredded
1 tablespoon salsa (optional)

For Dessert
1 medium orange

Instructions: Lightly coat a large nonstick sauté pan with vegetable spray, and heat over medium flame. Add onion and green pepper and sauté, stirring often, until tender, about 10 minutes. Remove and set aside. Meanwhile, beat egg whites with milk, if desired. Stir in chili powder. Heat olive oil in the large nonstick sauté pan over medium heat. Pour in the egg whites and cook until almost set, occasionally lifting edges so that uncooked portion flows underneath, 2 to 3 minutes. When eggs are set, place onions, green pepper, black beans, and cheese on top. Fold with a spatula and continue cooking until lightly browned, about 1 minute. Top with salsa. Serve orange for dessert.

*No one wants to chop vegetables first thing in the morning. Buy a bag of frozen onions and green peppers and just pour out what you need. Return the rest to the freezer.

Lunch: Grilled Chicken Salad

Ingredients
1 cup green-leaf or romaine lettuce, washed, dried, and torn into large pieces
1 cup broccoli florets
½ green pepper, cored, seeded, and cut into thin strips
1 medium tomato, sliced
1 tablespoon olive oil-and-vinegar dressing*
1 tablespoon lemon juice
1 teaspoon Worcestershire sauce
½ teaspoon freshly ground pepper, or to taste
3 ounces precooked grilled skinless chicken breast, sliced into bite-sized chunks

For Dessert
1 medium pear

Instructions: Toss lettuce with broccoli, green pepper, and tomato. Combine dressing with the lemon juice, Worcestershire sauce, and pepper. Toss with vegetables until well combined, and top with chicken chunks. Serve pear for dessert.

Zone oil-and-vinegar dressing contains 1 teaspoon olive oil and 2 teaspoons vinegar. Extra vinegar may be added to taste.

Dinner: Broiled Salmon

Ingredients
    4½ ounces salmon steak, about 1 inch thick
    1 teaspoon olive oil
    ½ teaspoon dried rosemary, or to taste
    ½ teaspoon dried tarragon, or to taste
    ½ teaspoon dried dill, or to taste
    2 cups zucchini, washed, ends removed, and sliced into ¼-inch
        strips

For Dessert
    1 apple

Instructions: Preheat broiler. Brush salmon with oil and sprinkle with herbs. On a roasting pan or aluminum foil, broil for 4–5 minutes per side, depending on thickness, turning once. Meanwhile, steam the zucchini: in a large pot fitted with a steaming basket, bring 1 inch water to boil. Add zucchini to the basket and steam until crisp-tender, 4 to 6 minutes. Serve apple for dessert.

Day 7

Breakfast: Vegetable Omelet

Ingredients
    1 cup asparagus spears, woody bases discarded, bias-sliced into
        1-inch pieces
    1 teaspoon olive oil
    ¼ cup yellow onions, peeled and finely chopped
    ½ cup button mushrooms, washed, dried, and thinly sliced

4 egg whites (or ½ cup egg substitute)
1 tablespoon low-fat milk (optional) vegetable spray
3 strips turkey bacon (substitute 1 ounce lean Canadian bacon
    or 2 soy sausage links)
⅔ cup mandarin oranges

Instructions: In a large pot fitted with a steaming basket, bring 1 inch water to boil. Add asparagus to the basket and steam until crisp-tender, 5 minutes, and set aside. Heat olive oil in a large non-stick sauté pan over medium heat. Add onions and mushrooms and lightly sauté until onion is wilted, about 10 minutes. Remove from pan and set aside to cool. Meanwhile, beat egg whites with milk, if desired. Stir in cooled onions and mushrooms. Lightly coat the sauté pan with vegetable spray, and heat over medium flame. Pour in the egg mixture and cook until almost set, occasionally lifting edges so that uncooked portion flows underneath, 2 to 3 minutes. When eggs are set, top with asparagus tips and fold with a spatula. Continue cooking until lightly browned, about 1 minute. Prepare bacon or soy links, following package instructions, and serve on the side with oranges.

Lunch: Stuffed Tomatoes

Ingredients
3 ounces albacore tuna packed in water, drained
1 tablespoon light mayonnaise
¼ cup celery, washed and minced
1 tablespoon onion, peeled and minced
2 large tomatoes, washed, tops removed, and hulled

For Dessert
1 nectarine

Instructions: In a medium mixing bowl, combine tuna, mayonnaise, celery, and onion. Stuff into tomatoes and serve. Serve nectarine for dessert.

Dinner: Chicken Marinara with Three-Bean Salad*

Ingredients

1½ cups green beans, washed, ends removed, and cut in half
¼ cup canned chickpeas, drained
¼ cup canned kidney beans, drained
1 teaspoon olive oil
2 tablespoons cider vinegar, or to taste
1 teaspoon dried chives
1 teaspoon dried parsley
½ teaspoon freshly ground pepper, or to taste
1½ teaspoons dried basil
2 ounces boneless, skinless chicken breast cutlets
2 tablespoons prepared tomato sauce
¼ teaspoon garlic powder, or to taste
1 ounce low-fat mozzarella cheese, shredded

If possible, make three-bean salad ahead of time (up to 2 days) and store, tightly sealed, in the refrigerator.

Instructions: Preheat oven to 450°. In a large pot fitted with a steaming basket, bring 1 inch water to boil. Add green beans to the basket and steam until crisp-tender, 10 minutes. Remove from basket, drain, and combine with chickpeas and kidney beans. In a small mixing bowl, combine olive oil, vinegar, chives, parsley, pepper, and 1 teaspoon of the basil; experiment with the oil-vinegar ratio to taste. Toss with beans, cover, and refrigerate for 30 minutes. Place chicken in a large piece of foil. Top chicken with tomato sauce and sprinkle with the remaining ½ teaspoon basil, garlic powder, and cheese. Fold foil loosely over chicken, leaving ample space for air. Carefully turn up and seal the ends and the middle so that juices won't leak out. Bake in the preheated oven for 20 minutes. Remove from oven and carefully open foil to prevent steam burns. Serve with bean salad.

TYPICAL MALE
Day 1

Breakfast: Fruit Salad

Ingredients
1 cup low-fat cottage cheese
1 cup fresh or reduced-sugar canned pineapple, cubed
⅔ cup reduced-sugar canned mandarin oranges, drained
4 macadamia nuts, crushed

Instructions: Place cottage cheese in a bowl. Fold in pineapple, oranges, and nuts.

Lunch: Chef's Salad

Ingredients
1 cup green-leaf lettuce (substitute lettuce of your choice), washed, dried, and torn into large pieces
½ cup canned chickpeas, drained and rinsed
½ cup button mushrooms, washed, dried, and coarsely chopped
½ cup celery, washed, dried, and coarsely chopped
4 teaspoons olive-oil-and-vinegar dressing*
3 ounces deli-style turkey breast, cut into strips
1½ ounces deli-style ham, cut into strips
1 ounce reduced-fat Swiss cheese (substitute any reduced-fat cheese), julienned

For Dessert
1 medium apple

Instructions: Toss lettuce with chickpeas, mushrooms, and celery. Dress, toss, and add meat and cheese. Serve apple for dessert.

Zone oil-and-vinegar dressing for this meal contains 1⅓ teaspoons olive oil and 2 teaspoons vinegar. Extra vinegar may be added to taste.

Dinner: Ginger Chicken

Ingredients
1⅓ teaspoons olive oil
4 ounces boneless, skinless chicken breast, cut lengthwise into
    thin strips
2 cups broccoli florets, washed
1½ cups snow peas, washed
¾ cup yellow onion, peeled and chopped
1 teaspoon fresh ginger, grated

For Dessert
1 cup seedless grapes

Instructions: In a wok or large nonstick pan, heat oil over medium-high heat. Add chicken and sauté, turning frequently, until lightly browned, about 5 minutes. Add broccoli, snow peas, onion, ginger, and ¼ cup water. Continue cooking, stirring often, until the chicken is done, water is reduced to a glaze, and vegetables are tender, about 20 minutes. If the pan dries out during cooking, add water in tablespoon increments to keep moist. Serve grapes for dessert.

Day 2

Breakfast: Yogurt and Fruit

Ingredients
1 ounce lean Canadian bacon (substitute 3 turkey bacon strips or
    2 soy sausage links)
½ cup fresh blueberries, rinsed and drained
4 teaspoons slivered almonds
1½ cups plain low-fat yogurt

Instructions: Prepare bacon or soy patties, following package instructions. Stir fruit and nuts into yogurt, and serve with bacon or links on the side.

Lunch: Tuna Salad

Ingredients

4 ounces albacore tuna packed in water, drained
¼ cup celery, washed, dried, and coarsely chopped
4 teaspoons olive-oil-and-vinegar dressing*
1 or 2 lettuce leaves, washed and dried
½ cantaloupe, seeds scooped out
¾ cup blueberries, rinsed and drained

Instructions: Mix tuna with celery and stir in dressing. Prepare a bed of the lettuce, and top with tuna mixture. Stuff cantaloupe with berries and serve for dessert.

Zone oil-and-vinegar dressing for this meal contains 1⅓ teaspoons olive oil and 2 teaspoons vinegar. Extra vinegar may be added to taste.

Dinner: Foiled Flounder with Green Beans

Ingredients

vegetable spray
6 ounces boneless flounder fillet (substitute mild, flaky fish of your choice)
2 tablespoons yellow onion, peeled and chopped
sprinkling of Parmesan cheese
¼ teaspoon freshly ground pepper, or to taste
squirt lemon juice
3 cups fresh green beans, washed, ends removed, and halved
4 teaspoons almonds, slivered

For Dessert

pineapple

Instructions: Preheat oven to 425°. Tear off an 18-inch-by-12-inch piece of foil. Spray the center lightly with vegetable spray, and place fish in the center of the foil. Top with onion and sprinkle with cheese, pepper, and lemon juice. Fold foil loosely over fish, leaving ample space for air. Carefully turn up and seal the ends and the middle so that juices won't leak out. Bake in the preheated oven 18 minutes. Meanwhile, steam the green beans: in a large pot fitted with a steaming basket, bring 1 inch water to boil. Add beans to the basket and steam until crisp-tender, 10 minutes. Drain, place in serving bowl, and fold in almonds. When fish is done, carefully open foil to prevent steam burns, and remove to a plate. Serve with green beans. Serve pineapple for dessert.

Day 3

Breakfast: Fruit Smoothie

Ingredients
    27 grams protein powder
    1¼ cup blueberries
    1½ cup strawberries
    4 macadamia nuts
    6 ice cubes

Instructions: Place all ingredients in a blender and blend at high speed until smooth, about 1 minute. Add a little water if smoothie is too thick. If you prefer, eat the nuts on the side.

Lunch: Cheeseburger

Ingredients
    4½ ounces lean (less than 10%) ground beef (substitute 4½ ounces ground turkey or 1½ soy burger patties)
    1 ounce reduced-fat American cheese (substitute cheese of choice)
    1 tablespoon light mayonnaise
    ½ hamburger roll
    1 thick tomato slice, optional
    1 large lettuce leaf, optional
    1 dill pickle wedge, optional
    3 black olives

For Dessert
1 cup unsweetened applesauce
sprinkling of cinnamon

Instructions: Preheat broiler. Place burger on foil or rack and broil 5 minutes. Flip and continue cooking another 5 minutes for medium rare. One minute before expected doneness, top with cheese, and remove when melted. Spread mayonnaise on the roll. Top with burger, tomato, and lettuce. Serve pickle on the side. Either chop olives and place on top of cheeseburger or serve them on the side. Sprinkle applesauce with cinnamon and serve for dessert.

Dinner: Vegetarian Stir-fry

Ingredients
1⅓ teaspoons olive oil
1 cup vegetable protein crumbles* (substitute 6 ounces firm tofu)
1½ cups yellow onions, peeled chopped
2 cups broccoli florets, washed
2 cups button mushrooms, washed, dried, and thinly sliced
1 ounce reduced-fat Swiss cheese, shredded

Morningstar Farms makes Burger Style Recipe Crumbles, which looks like ground beef and is a good vegetarian source of protein.

For Dessert
1 cup grapes

Instructions: Heat oil in a nonstick sauté pan or wok over medium-high heat. If using tofu, remove from wrapping, drain, and crumble. Add tofu or soy crumbles and stir until mixed with the oil. Add onions, broccoli, and mushrooms. Reduce heat to medium and stir-fry, stirring often, until vegetables are tender, about 15 minutes. Stir in cheese and heat until melted, about 1 minute. Serve grapes for dessert.

Day 4

Breakfast: Scrambled Eggs and Bacon

Ingredients
vegetable spray
6 egg whites (or ¾ cup egg substitute)
1⅓ teaspoons olive oil
1 tablespoon low-fat milk (optional)
1 ounce lean Canadian bacon (substitute 3 turkey bacon strips
    or 2 soy sausage links)

For Dessert
1 cup grapes
⅔ cup mandarin oranges

Instructions: Lightly coat a large nonstick pan with vegetable spray, and heat over medium flame. Beat egg whites with olive oil and milk, if desired. Pour into pan and cook, stirring often, until scrambled and fully set. Prepare bacon or soy links, following package instructions. Mix grapes and oranges and serve for dessert.

Lunch: Tofu Dip and Veggies

Ingredients
6 ounces firm tofu
1 ounce reduced-fat Swiss cheese, grated
½ cup canned chickpeas, drained and rinsed
1⅓ teaspoons olive oil
2 tablespoons fresh lemon juice
2 tablespoons Lipton dry onion soup mix (substitute spices of
    your choice, to taste*)
1 medium green pepper, washed, cored, seeded, and cut in
    wedges
2 cups broccoli florets

For Dessert
1 kiwi

Instructions: Drain tofu. Put tofu, cheese, chickpeas, olive oil, lemon juice, and onion soup mix in a blender. Blend until smooth. (For best flavor, refrigerate the dip at least 2 hours or overnight.) Place dip in a bowl in the center of a large plate. Arrange pepper strips and broccoli around bowl for dipping. Serve kiwi for dessert.

*If you don't want to use the packaged soup mix, experiment with minced onions, garlic, or vegetable bouillon granules.

Dinner: Spiced Lamb with Vegetables

Ingredients
6 ounces lean ground lamb
⅕ cup brown rice
1 teaspoon cider vinegar
1⅓ teaspoons olive oil
½ cup scallions, finely chopped
¾ cup red onions, chunks
2 cups mushrooms
1½ cups tomatoes, diced
½ cup green beans, diced
1 tablespoon cilantro
2 teaspoons fresh ginger, minced
¼ teaspoon cumin
¼ teaspoon coriander
⅛ teaspoon black pepper
½ teaspoon celery salt
⅛ teaspoon cinnamon

Instructions: In a small glass bowl, combine lamb, rice, vinegar, and spices. Cover and refrigerate for 30 minutes. Heat the oil in a medium nonstick sauté pan. Add meat mixture and vegetables. Cook, breaking meat up as it cooks, until lamb is cooked through and vegetables are tender. Spoon onto plate and serve.

Day 5

Breakfast: Old-Fashioned Oatmeal

Ingredients

1 cup slow-cooking (steel-cut) oatmeal*
2 ounces lean Canadian bacon (substitute 6 turkey bacon strips
     or 1 soy sausage patty)
⅓ cup unsweetened applesauce
1 tablespoon almonds, slivered
sprinkling of nutmeg
sprinkling of cinnamon
½ cup low-fat cottage cheese

Instructions: Bring 3 cups water to a brisk boil over high heat. Add oatmeal, stirring well. When smooth and beginning to thicken, reduce heat to low and simmer for 30 minutes, stirring occasionally. While oatmeal is cooking, prepare bacon or soy patties, following package instructions. Remove oatmeal from the heat. Stir in apple-sauce and almonds. Sprinkle with cinnamon and nutmeg. Serve bacon and cottage cheese on the side.

*By slow cooking, we mean slow *cooking. Oatmeal that calls itself slow-cooking but takes only 5 minutes isn't the real McCoy (or perhaps we should say the real McCann's, a popular brand). To shorten the morning cooking time, make a big batch during the weekend, freeze, and microwave the correct amount in the morning. You may also put the oatmeal in a wide-mouth thermos with 1⅓ cups boiling water, and let it cook overnight.*

Lunch: Chili (Meat or Vegetarian)

Ingredients

1⅓ teaspoons olive oil
6 ounces lean (less than 10%) ground beef (substitute ground
     turkey or 1⅓ cups vegetable protein crumbles*)
¼ cup yellow onions, peeled and minced

1 teaspoon chili powder, or to taste
½ teaspoon garlic powder, or to taste
½ teaspoon freshly ground pepper, or to taste
1½ cups salsa or stewed tomatoes with liquid
¼ cup kidney beans, drained and rinsed
       sprinkling of low-fat Monterey Jack cheese (optional)

Instructions: In a large nonstick sauté pan, heat oil over medium-high flame. Add meat and sauté, stirring often, until lightly browned, about 5 minutes. If using protein crumbles, heat until blended with oil, about 2 minutes. Add onions, chili powder, garlic powder, pepper, salsa, and kidney beans. Simmer, stirring occasionally, until onion is wilted and flavors are blended, about 20 minutes. Place in bowl and top with cheese, if desired.

*Morningstar Farms makes Burger Style Recipe Crumbles, which looks like ground beef and is a good vegetarian source of protein.

Dinner: Shrimp Scampi with Vegetables

Ingredients
1⅓ teaspoons olive oil
1½ cups asparagus spears, washed, woody bases discarded, and
       bias-sliced into 1-inch-long pieces
1½ cups yellow onions, peeled and finely chopped
1 medium green pepper, washed, cored, seeded, and roughly
       chopped
2 cloves garlic, peeled and minced, or to taste
6 ounces shrimp, shelled and deveined
¼ cup dry white wine (optional)
1–2 teaspoons lemon juice, or to taste
2 lemon wedges, optional

For Dessert
1 medium peach

Instructions: In a large nonstick pan, heat oil over medium-high heat. Sauté asparagus, onions, green pepper, and garlic, stirring often, until tender, about 10 minutes. Add shrimp, white wine, and lemon juice. Lower heat to medium and cook 5 minutes, stirring often, until shrimp are pink. Place on plate and garnish with lemon wedges. Serve peach for dessert.

Day 6

Breakfast: Spanish Omelet

Ingredients
vegetable spray
2 tablespoons yellow onion, peeled and finely chopped*
2 tablespoons green pepper, cored, seeded, and roughly chopped*
6 large egg whites (or ¾ cup egg substitute)
1 tablespoon low-fat milk (optional)
1 teaspoon chili powder, or to taste (optional)
1⅓ teaspoons olive oil
½ cup canned black beans, drained
1 ounce low-fat Monterey Jack cheese, shredded
1 tablespoon salsa (optional)

For Dessert
1 medium orange

Instructions: Lightly coat a large nonstick sauté pan with vegetable spray, and heat over medium flame. Add onion and green pepper and sauté, stirring often, until tender, about 10 minutes. Remove and set aside. Meanwhile, beat egg whites with milk, if desired. Stir in chili powder. Heat olive oil in the large nonstick sauté pan over medium heat. Pour in the egg whites and cook until almost set, occasionally lifting edges so that uncooked portion flows underneath, 2 to 3 minutes. When eggs are set, place onions, green pepper, black beans, and cheese on top. Fold with a spatula and continue cooking until lightly browned, about 1 minute. Top with salsa. Serve orange for dessert.

No one wants to chop vegetables first thing in the morning. Buy a bag of frozen onions and green peppers and just pour out what you need. Return the rest to the freezer.

Lunch: Grilled Chicken Salad

Ingredients
2 cups green-leaf or romaine lettuce, washed, dried, and torn into large pieces
1 cup broccoli florets
½ green pepper, cored, seeded, and cut into thin strips
¼ cup canned kidney beans, rinsed and drained
1 medium tomato, sliced
4 teaspoons olive oil-and-vinegar dressing*
1 tablespoon lemon juice
1 teaspoon Worcestershire sauce
½ teaspoon freshly ground pepper, or to taste
4 ounces precooked grilled skinless chicken breast, sliced into bite-sized chunks

For Dessert
1 medium pear

Instructions: Toss lettuce with broccoli, green pepper, kidney beans, and tomato. Combine dressing with the lemon juice, Worcestershire sauce, and pepper. Toss with vegetables until well combined, and top with chicken chunks. Serve pear for dessert.

**Zone oil-and-vinegar dressing for this meal contains 1⅓ teaspoons olive oil and 2 teaspoons vinegar. Extra vinegar may be added to taste.*

Dinner: Broiled Salmon

Ingredients
6 ounces salmon steak, about 1 inch thick
1⅓ teaspoons olive oil
½ teaspoon dried rosemary, or to taste
½ teaspoon dried tarragon, or to taste

½ teaspoon dried dill, or to taste

2 cups zucchini, washed, ends removed, and sliced into ¼-inch
strips

For Dessert
1 apple
1 plum

Instructions: Preheat broiler. Brush salmon with olive oil and sprinkle with herbs. On a roasting pan or aluminum foil, broil for 4–5 minutes per side, depending on thickness, turning once. Meanwhile, steam the zucchini: in a large pot fitted with a steaming basket, bring 1 inch water to boil. Add zucchini to the basket and steam until crisp-tender, 4 to 6 minutes. Serve apple and plum for dessert.

Day 7

Breakfast: Vegetable Omelet

Ingredients
1 cup asparagus spears, woody bases discarded, bias-sliced into
1-inch pieces
1⅓ teaspoons olive oil
¼ cup yellow onions, peeled and finely chopped
½ cup button mushrooms, washed, dried, and thinly sliced
6 egg whites (or ¾ cup egg substitute)
1 tablespoon low-fat milk (optional)
vegetable spray
3 strips turkey bacon (substitute 1 ounce lean Canadian bacon
or 2 soy sausage links)
1 cup mandarin oranges

Instructions: In a large pot fitted with a steaming basket, bring 1 inch water to boil. Add asparagus to the basket and steam until crisp-tender, 5 minutes, and set aside. Heat olive oil in a large non-stick sauté pan over medium heat. Add onions and mushrooms and lightly sauté until onion is wilted, about 10 minutes. Remove from pan and set aside to cool. Meanwhile, beat egg whites with milk, if desired. Stir in cooled onions and mushrooms. Lightly coat the sauté pan with vegetable spray, and heat over medium flame. Pour in the egg mixture and cook until almost set, occasionally lifting edges so that uncooked portion flows underneath, 2 to 3 minutes. When eggs are set, top with asparagus tips and fold with a spatula. Continue cooking until lightly browned, about 1 minute. Prepare bacon or soy links, following package instructions, and serve on the side with oranges.

Lunch: Stuffed Tomatoes

Ingredients
　　4 ounces albacore tuna packed in water, drained
　　4 teaspoons light mayonnaise
　　¼ cup celery, washed and minced
　　1 tablespoon onion, peeled and minced
　　2 large tomatoes, washed, tops removed, and hulled
　　1 small bread stick

For Dessert
　　1 nectarine

Instructions: In a medium mixing bowl, combine tuna, mayonnaise, celery, and onion. Stuff into tomatoes and serve. Serve bread stick on the side. Serve nectarine for dessert.

Dinner: Chicken Marinara with Three-Bean Salad*

Ingredients
　　1½ cups green beans, washed, ends removed, and cut in half
　　¼ cup canned chickpeas, drained
　　¼ cup canned kidney beans, drained
　　1⅓ teaspoons olive oil

If possible, make the three-bean salad ahead of time (up to 2 days) and store, tightly sealed, in refrigerator.

2 tablespoons cider vinegar, or to taste

1 teaspoon dried chives

1 teaspoon dried parsley

½ teaspoon freshly ground pepper, or to taste

1½ teaspoons dried basil

3 ounces boneless, skinless chicken breast cutlets

2 tablespoons prepared tomato sauce

¼ teaspoon garlic powder, or to taste

1 ounce low-fat mozzarella cheese, shredded

For Dessert

1 peach

Instructions: Preheat oven to 450°. In a large pot fitted with a steaming basket, bring 1 inch water to boil. Add green beans to the basket and steam until crisp-tender, 10 minutes. Remove from basket, drain, and combine with chickpeas and kidney beans. In a small mixing bowl, combine olive oil, vinegar, chives, parsley, pepper, and 1 teaspoon of the basil; experiment with the oil-vinegar ratio to taste. Toss with beans, cover, and refrigerate for 30 minutes. Place chicken in a large piece of foil. Top chicken with tomato sauce and sprinkle with the remaining ½ teaspoon basil, garlic powder, and cheese. Fold foil loosely over chicken, leaving ample space for air. Carefully turn up and seal the ends and the middle so that juices won't leak out. Bake in the preheated oven for 20 minutes. Remove from oven and carefully open foil to prevent steam burns. Serve with bean salad. Serve peach for dessert.

6

MORE QUICK AND EASY ZONE BREAKFASTS, LUNCHES, DINNERS, AND SNACKS

Once you have spent a week in the Zone enjoying the meals provided in Chapter 5, I'm confident that you'll want to continue improving your health and appearance by eating more Zone meals. However, I also realize that finding the time to prepare healthy, appetizing meals can be something of a challenge. Therefore, all the recipes in this chapter are not only guaranteed to keep you in the Zone, they are also designed to minimize your time and effort in the kitchen. By combining these meals with those already offered in Chapter 5, you'll have a great set of breakfasts, lunches, dinners, and snacks to choose from every day.

Whereas all of the recipes in Chapter 5 were broken down into recipes for men and recipes for women, in this section, all of the recipes are calculated to fit into the male requirements. Does this mean you can't eat the recipes if you're a woman? Of course not—simply prepare the recipe as directed, then set aside ¼ of the finished dish, and save it as a snack for later. Better yet, simply reduce the recipe by ¼ before cooking. This may seem complicated, but remember that the Zone does not need to be an exact science. Take away a bit of the protein, carbohydrates, and fat, and you'll have a meal that fits perfectly into your unique eating plan.

All recipes make one serving.

BREAKFASTS

Blueberry Pancakes

Ingredients
1 whole egg
1⅓ cups soy flour*
1 cup 1% milk
½ teaspoon vanilla
½ teaspoon cinnamon
½ cup blueberries
1⅓ teaspoons olive oil

Instructions: In a small mixing bowl, combine eggs, soy flour, milk, ⅔ teaspoon olive oil, vanilla, cinnamon, and blueberries to form a thin batter. Heat ⅔ teaspoon oil in a nonstick sauté pan. Pour batter into pan to make small (2-inch) pancakes. Batter will make about 24 silver-dollar-sized pancakes. The pancakes will cook to a golden brown and will resemble buckwheat pancakes in color and flavor. As pancakes are cooked, place on two serving plates and keep warm. Repeat process until all batter is used.

Available in some health food stores.

French Toast Sticks

Ingredients
1 slice whole-grain bread
4 large egg whites or ½ cup egg substitute
vegetable spray
confectioners' sugar
1 cup strawberries, sliced
1 tablespoon slivered almonds
1 ounce extra-lean Canadian bacon or 3 slices turkey bacon

Instructions: Cut bread into sticks and soak in beaten eggs. (Scramble any egg mixture that remains.) Spray a nonstick pan with vegetable spray. Over medium-low heat, cook bread sticks, turning often until done. Roll cooked bread sticks in a little bit of confectioners' sugar. Top with sliced strawberries and slivered almonds. Cook bacon and serve on the side.

Huevos Rancheros

Ingredients
1⅓ teaspoons olive oil
1 whole egg
2 egg whites
chopped onion, green pepper, and tomato
chili powder to taste
1 corn tortilla
2 ounces low-fat cheese
1 tablespoon chopped cilantro

Side Dish
1 cup honeydew melon, cubed

Instructions: Heat oil in skillet. Scramble egg, egg whites, chopped vegetables, and chili powder. Place scrambled eggs in tortilla and top with cheese and cilantro. Roll up tortilla.

Oatmeal

1 cup cooked oatmeal fortified with 2 tablespoons (1 ounce) protein powder (always add the protein powder after cooking the oatmeal).

Bagel and Lox

1 small plain bagel, 3 ounces lox or smoked salmon, and 3 tablespoons of light cream cheese.

LUNCHES

Turkey or Tuna Sandwich

4 ounces turkey breast or tuna with 1 teaspoon mayonnaise and 2 pieces of whole-rye bread.

Seafood Salad

Ingredients
  4½ ounces seafood (shrimp, crab meat, lobster)
  1 teaspoon light mayonnaise
  1 mini-pita pocket or 1 piece rye bread*

For Dessert
  ½ orange

Instructions: Mix seafood and mayonnaise. Stuff in mini-pita pocket.

You may eliminate the bread and place the seafood on top of a tossed salad. If you use the mayonnaise with the seafood, don't use salad dressing. Or substitute 1 tablespoon olive oil and vinegar dressing and hold the mayonnaise.

Tomato-Basil Salad

Ingredients
  5 cups romaine lettuce, chopped
  ¼ cup chickpeas, rinsed and finely chopped
  1 tablespoon fresh parsley, chopped
  1⅓ teaspoons olive oil
  1 tablespoon red wine vinegar
  2 tablespoons fresh basil, chopped
  1 teaspoon garlic, minced
  ¼ teaspoon chili powder

2 cups tomatoes, sliced
4 ounces skim-milk mozzarella cheese, shredded

For Dessert
1 apple or pear
½ cup strawberries

Instructions: Place lettuce on a serving plate. In a medium bowl, combine chickpeas, parsley, oil, vinegar, basil, garlic, and chili powder. Alternate slices of tomato and shredded mozzarella on the lettuce bed. Pour chickpea dressing over tomatoes and serve. Eat fruit for dessert.

BLT Sandwich

Ingredients
1 slice rye bread
2 ounces lean Canadian bacon
3 leaves lettuce
2 tomato slices
1 ounce low-fat cheese
1 teaspoon light mayonnaise

Side Dishes
½ orange
12 peanuts

Picnic-style Cold Tempeh Salad

Ingredients
4 ounces tempeh, cubed
1 tablespoon tamari sauce
1½ tablespoons mayonnaise
¼ cup plain yogurt
juice of ½ lemon

2 teaspoons prepared mustard
3 medium celery stalks
1 medium green pepper, diced
3 hard-boiled egg whites
1 slice red onion, diced
3 black olives, sliced
1 sprig fresh dill or parsley, minced

Instructions: Preheat oven to 350°. Toss tempeh with tamari sauce in baking dish and bake uncovered for 10 to 12 minutes. Set aside to cool. Mix mayonnaise, yogurt, lemon juice, and mustard. Add celery, green pepper, egg whites, and red onion. Fold in tempeh cubes and sprinkle with olives and herbs. Chill and serve on a bed of lettuce, if desired.

DINNERS

Grilled Sole with Leeks

Ingredients
1⅓ teaspoons olive oil
3 cups sliced leeks
6 ounces fillet of sole
4 ounces white wine (optional)
1 teaspoon minced garlic
1 shallot, minced
1 teaspoon dill
salt to taste
pepper to taste
½ teaspoon lemon herb seasoning

Instructions: Preheat oven to 375°. Brush a medium baking dish with the olive oil. Layer bottom of dish with leeks. Place sole on top. In a medium bowl, combine wine, garlic, shallots, dill, salt, and pepper. Gently pour wine mixture into baking dish. Sprinkle with lemon herb seasoning. Tightly cover baking dish and place in oven. Bake for 25 to 30 minutes and serve.

Pork Medallions and Apples

Ingredients
3 ounces pork medallions or thinly sliced pork chops
½ apple
rosemary to taste
Dijon mustard to taste
1 to 2 tablespoons white wine (optional)
¼ cup water

Side Dishes
1 cup cooked broccoli
1 spinach salad with dressing (1 tablespoon olive oil and vinegar to taste)

Instructions: Preheat oven to 450°. Place pork in a baking dish in a single layer. Top with apple slices, rosemary, and mustard. Pour wine and water around the pork. Bake for 15 minutes. Baste pork with pan juices. Reduce heat to 350° and continue cooking for 10 to 15 minutes, until pork is white, not pink, inside.

Chicken Fajitas

Ingredients
4 ounces boneless chicken breast
2 tablespoons salsa
2 tablespoons bottled lime juice
salt to taste
freshly ground black pepper to taste
¼ cup water or more
⅓ green pepper, cut into quarters, seeds and membrane removed
⅓ red pepper, cut into quarters, seeds and membrane removed
⅓ yellow onion, sliced into ¼-inch-wide rings, and microwaved on high for 2 minutes, stirring after 1 minute
1 fajita-size (8") tortilla

Condiments

½ cup chopped tomato

1⅓ tablespoons guacamole

For Dessert

½ cup strawberries

Instructions: Slice chicken breasts crosswise into ½-inch strips. Place in a glass dish with salsa, lime juice, salt, and pepper and enough water to cover. Cover with plastic wrap and refrigerate overnight. Into a large skillet, over high heat, pour in the liquid from the chicken and cook to reduce by half. Add the chicken strips and, using a wide wooden spatula, toss frequently. When chicken turns opaque but is not yet thoroughly cooked, add the peppers and onion. Continue cooking and tossing the mixture. Cook until the liquid has evaporated and it begins to sizzle. Give one more toss and remove from heat. Serve with tortilla and condiments.

Cioppino

Ingredients

1⅓ teaspoons olive oil

¾ cup chopped onion

1 cup chopped green pepper

1½ cups chopped canned tomatoes

4 cups chopped mushrooms

1 teaspoon minced garlic

1 tablespoon parsley, chopped

¼ teaspoon dried oregano

¼ teaspoon dried basil

⅛ teaspoon cayenne pepper

salt to taste

pepper to taste

½ cup lemon- and lime-flavored water

4 ounces dry red wine (optional)

1½ ounces cherrystone clams

1½ ounces sole
1½ ounces small shrimp, shelled and deveined
1½ ounces baby bay scallops

Instructions: In a medium saucepan, combine oil, vegetables, spices, water, and wine. Bring to a boil, reduce heat, and bring to a simmer. Add seafood, cover, and simmer for 5 to 7 minutes. Spoon into a bowl and serve.

Tofu-Vegetable Kebabs with Yogurt Olive Dip

Ingredients

¼ cup plain low-fat yogurt
3 black olives, sliced
2 teaspoons prepared mustard
1 teaspoon honey
½ teaspoon light miso
1 sprig fresh parsley, minced
2 medium zucchini, cubed
1 large onion, cut into small chunks
7 ounces extra-firm tofu, cubed
12 whole mushrooms
6 cherry tomatoes
1 teaspoon olive oil
salt to taste
pepper to taste

Instructions: Mix yogurt, olives, mustard, honey, miso, and parsley. Set aside. Blanch zucchini and onion in boiling water for two minutes, then drain. Onion may separate, which is to be expected. Alternate tofu, zucchini, onion, mushrooms, and cherry tomatoes on skewers, always ending with a mushroom. Brush with olive oil and salt and pepper lightly. Place under broiler or on outdoor grill. Turn after 5 minutes and grill another 5 minutes. Serve with yogurt-olive dip.

Snacks

- 2 hard-boiled egg whites, cut in half and stuffed with ¼ cup hummus
- 1 ounce low-fat string cheese
- ½ cup grapes
- 3 olives
- 1½ ounces deli-style turkey
- ½ apple
- 3 peanuts
- ¼ cup low-fat cottage cheese
- ½ cup pineapple
- 1 teaspoon slivered almonds
- 1 ounce cheese
- 4 ounces wine
- 1 cup 1% milk
- 3 macadamia nuts
- 1 Wasa cracker
- 1 ounce low-fat cheese
- 3 sliced olives (zap for 10 seconds in the microwave)
- 2 ounces firm tofu
- ⅓ teaspoon olive oil
- sprinkling of Lipton dry onion soup mix
- ⅛ cup chickpeas (blend until smooth)
- 1 sliced green pepper for dipping

Frozen Meals

The following frozen meals can fit into the Zone, but sometimes need a little tinkering. Therefore, read the food labels carefully.

Stouffer's Lean Cuisine
Beef Peppercorn
Grilled Chicken
Chicken and Vegetables

Healthy Choice
Grilled Chicken Sonoma (sprinkle a little Parmesan cheese on top)

Grilled Peppercorn Beef Patty
Garlic Chicken Milano (sprinkle a little Parmesan cheese on top)
Turkey Breast Medallions (add 2 teaspoons slivered almonds
    and have ¼ cup grapes for dessert)

Marie Callender
Grilled Turkey Breast Strips
Swedish Meatballs (a little high in fat)

Weight Watchers (these meals need quite a bit of work to get them into the Zone)
Fiesta Chicken (add 2 teaspoons slivered almonds and either 1
    ounce low-fat cheese or 1 additional ounce of chicken)
Creamy Rigatoni with Broccoli Chicken (add 2 ounces chicken
    and 9 sliced olives)

7

DINING OUT IN THE ZONE

Americans are eating out like never before. At least 50 percent of all meals are now eaten outside the home. Once you master preparing Zone meals at home, transferring that knowledge to the outside world is very easy.

What is the easiest (but the most expensive) way of dining out in the Zone? Go to a very expensive French restaurant. For around fifty dollars, you'll get a glass of great wine and a small amount of protein (no bigger and no thicker than the palm of your hand) surrounded by an artistically arranged outer ring of vegetables with a small side salad to cleanse the palate. And for dessert you'll have some fresh fruit. But the key to gourmet French cooking is the sauce, which is composed of fat. This is why most nutritionists hate the French: they eat too much fat, they smoke, they drink, and they don't exercise. But their biggest complaint about the French is that they seem to enjoy themselves. On the other hand, it's difficult to ignore the fact that the French have the lowest rate of heart disease in Europe, and they look good in designer clothing.

No one has ever accused the French of not eating well, but you now realize that a gourmet French meal is really a Zone·meal. A gourmet French meal contains adequate (but not excessive) amounts of protein, lots of low-density vegetables, a little fruit for dessert, and a glass of wine (which the body treats like a carbohydrate) to balance off the protein. A little fat in the sauce not only adds to the taste, but also slows down the rate of entry of carbohydrates into the bloodstream.

Okay, eating at four-star French restaurants is a pretty expensive way to eat out in the Zone, since you could have had five meals at the all-you-can-eat pasta palace for the same price. But how do you stay in the Zone when you're going out to a typical restaurant, where a satisfied customer is one who has to unbuckle his belt after the meal? Here are some simple rules to follow at any restaurant, four-star or family-style.

Rule #1. Never eat the rolls. If you're going to eat carbohydrates, save it for dessert. Isn't that the reason you went to restaurant in the first place? More about this later.

Rule #2. Always choose your low-fat protein entree from the menu first, before you order anything else. This sets the stage for ordering the rest of your meal. Then ask the waiter to replace any starches or grains with extra vegetables.

Rule #3. While you're waiting for dinner, have a glass of red wine or a glass of bottled water while everyone else is munching on their rolls. Try conversation instead of eating to pass the time.

Rule #4. Once the dinner is served, look at the size of the low-fat protein entree you ordered. If it is significantly greater in size than the palm of your hand, plan to take the excess home (it sure beats eating cottage cheese the next day). Then look at your plate and determine whether the carbohydrates are favorable or unfavorable.

Rule #5. The volume of the low-fat protein you plan to eat determines the volume of the carbohydrate you are going to eat. If you're eating favorable carbohydrates, then plan to have double the volume of carbohydrates compared to the protein portion.

Rule #6. If you really came to the restaurant to eat dessert, then don't eat any carbohydrates at the meal. The waiter will still take your plate away. When he or she comes back with a dessert menu, order whatever you want, but plan to only eat half. The rest of the dessert? Offer it to your dinner companions. I'm sure they will be delighted to help out. Of course, if you want to eat a full dessert, have fresh fruit just like the French do.

Now that wasn't too difficult. This is very easy to do in the four-star French restaurant, where there isn't very much food to begin with, but much more difficult to undertake at the typical restaurant, where massive volumes of food are pushed in your direction. And this is what has happened to American restaurants in the last generation. Because we have the cheapest food on earth, people expect to get their money's worth by consuming massive amounts of calories. Everything is oversized. The only exceptions are the exclusive (and expensive) restaurants, where presentation and quality count far more than sheer bulk. And since mass is in, you make your money as a restaurant owner by making sure most of the food volume comes in the form of carbohydrates (which are cheap) as opposed to protein (which is relatively expensive).

THE FAST FOOD ZONE

It's just as easy to make hormonally correct meals in fast food restaurants, if you remember the Zone rules. Let's take McDonald's, for example. Here's a very quick meal. Buy the grilled McChicken sandwich and a salad. Throw away three-quarters of the bun, add the grilled chicken and one-quarter of the bun to the salad, and presto, you have a grilled chicken salad with a large crouton. It's quick, it's easy, and it's hormonally correct if you know the rules. Fast food restaurants can be a great help for those times when you don't have the time to cook or sit at a restaurant because they always have protein (unfortunately, much of it is high-fat hamburgers, so always try to choose the chicken entrees). The secret of fast food in the Zone is knowing when to stop adding carbohydrates. Some of the Zone meals that can be found in fast food restaurants are shown below.

Fast Food Zone Meals

Wendy's
   12 oz. of chili

McDonald's
   Grilled McChicken Sandwich (throw away ¼ of the bun)

Burger King
   BK Broiler without mayo (throw away ¼ of the bun)

Taco Bell

Chicken tacos

However, the best fast food meals can be found in your supermarket at the salad bar. Simply grab a bunch of precut vegetables and fruits (especially the things you would never buy otherwise), and put them in the tin plate they provide, along with some olives (your monounsaturated fat). Then walk over to the deli and buy a quarter-pound of low-fat protein, such as turkey, chicken, or tuna. Add the low-fat protein to your precut vegetables, fruits, and olives, and you've got a great Zone meal. It may be a little expensive compared to a bagel and a cup of coffee, but isn't your health worth it?

ZONE MEALS FOR THE BUSINESS TRAVELER

How do you stay in the Zone if you are constantly on the road? Here are some easy tricks. If you are staying for a couple of days at a hotel that has a room refrigerator, then go out and buy some fruit and sliced low-fat deli meat or low-fat cottage cheese. For every piece of fruit, plan to eat 1 ounce of low-fat meat or 2 ounces of cottage cheese. These can be quick snacks before you go out to eat (thereby making it easier to stay in the Zone at the restaurant) for the times you can't prepare your own food. And before you go to bed, have a quick Zone snack as a hormonal "touch-up" so that you get a good night's sleep in a strange bed.

Keep in mind that Zone meals are your key to business success on the road, because they will determine your mental alertness throughout the day. Listed in the table below are some of the Zone winners that will give you an unfair advantage over your competitors. And, of course, never eat the rolls. Life is tough enough on the road without wandering out of the Zone.

Zone Meals for the Business Traveler

Breakfast

6-egg-white omelet plus oatmeal (don't eat the toast or the potatoes)

Breakfast buffet with scrambled eggs and fruit or scrambled
eggs and oatmeal (but choose only one)

Lunch

Grilled chicken Caesar salad with extra side of vegetables and
fresh fruit for dessert

Dinner

Fish with extra vegetables and no starches (that also means no
rolls) and fresh fruit for dessert

Holidays

During the Christmas season, the average American gains 5 to
10 pounds. Not so in the Zone. In fact, the typical holiday buffet
gives you an excellent opportunity to make great Zone meals. When
you are going through the buffet, always look for the low-fat protein first, and then just follow the eye and palm method outlined
earlier. Make sure that most of your carbohydrates come from vegetables and fruits, and try the best you can to ignore the grains,
breads, rolls, bagels, and pasta that usually characterize holiday
entertaining.

Holidays also usually mean alcohol consumption. Since the
body treats alcohol like a carbohydrate, always plan to have a protein chaser with every drink. An example might be a glass of wine
with a piece of soft cheese, or a bottle of beer with six cocktail
shrimp. Just make sure that you eat all the necessary protein before
your next drink. Again, it's a matter of balance.

In summary, eating out in the Zone is easy, if you know the
rules. "Just say no" to the overwhelming incoming tide of carbohydrates you're constantly exposed to when eating out. If you think
it's difficult, then think of carbohydrates as a drug. The more you
take of any drug, the more likely you are to suffer from a drug over-
dose. In this case, it's an excess production of insulin, which can
cause your premature death. That thought should make it easier to
pass on the rolls.

8

THE SOY ZONE

A very common confusion about the Zone is that you must eat animal protein to follow the program. Nothing could be further from the truth. To stay in the Zone only requires that you consume adequate protein. For vegans, the vegetarian version of the Zone uses vegetable sources of protein, primarily soy. Lacto-ovo vegetarians have an even greater protein variety because they can use low-fat egg products (such as egg whites) and low-fat dairy sources (cheeses, milk, and yogurt) in addition to soy products. However, as I describe in greater detail in my book *The Soy Zone*, the most powerful version of Zone that has the greatest potential health benefits uses primarily soy protein. Soy is an amazing food that everyone, whether a vegetarian or die-hard meat lover, should incorporate into their diet.

SOY: THE WONDER PROTEIN

Soybeans are unique because they are the only beans that contain slightly more protein than carbohydrate, and they contain certain phytochemicals known as isoflavones that have remarkable health benefits.

For a thousand years, the most widely available protein-rich source of soy protein was tofu. Many Americans are a bit wary of tofu, but it is actually an incredibly versatile food that easily absorbs flavor and can be used in a huge array of dishes. Now, with new technology, a great variety of soy meat substitutes that look and taste like meat products (hamburgers, sausages, and hot dogs) are also available. As a result, Americans are likely to begin making more soy-based meals.

The scientific data on the benefits of increased soy protein consumption is continually expanding. In fact, the FDA has recently allowed food manufacturers to make health claims about soy products and heart disease. Some of the benefits of increased soy consumption are listed below.

Health Benefits of Soy

Decreased cholesterol
Decreased heart disease
Decreased breast cancer
Decreased prostate cancer
Decreased osteoporosis
Decreased symptoms of menopause

Admittedly, many of these benefits come from epidemiological studies, which study large populations of people who eat soy, and then compare them to the similar populations that eat very little soy. But clinical studies do indicate one very unique distinguishing characteristic of soy protein: it lowers insulin and increases glucagon to a greater extent than does the same amount of animal protein. Since the goal of the Zone is to maintain insulin within a zone, the increased use of soy protein in your Zone meals, even if you're not a vegetarian, can be a very powerful tool for achieving that goal.

This unique hormonal property of improved insulin control, described in greater detail in *The Soy Zone*, accounts for many of the health benefits of soy protein. In addition, the isoflavones found in soy products also have the ability to alter the hormonal action of insulin. All in all, this makes soy protein one of the most beneficial foods you can eat in the Zone.

THE LONGEST-LIVED PEOPLE IN THE WORLD

I feel that one of the primary reasons for why a person changes eating patterns—whether that means entering the Zone or eating more soy protein—is to live a longer and better life. If that is the goal, then the best starting point for developing the ideal diet would be to study what the longest-lived people in the world actually eat.

It turns out the longest-lived people (with legitimate birth records to verify their ages) live on the Japanese island of Okinawa. Okinawans have a 40 percent lower mortality rate than the second longest-lived people, the mainland Japanese, and they have a greater percentage of centenarians (people living to 100) than any other country in the world. In fact, five times more Okinawans reach the age of 100 as mainland Japanese.

What accounts for the longevity of the Okinawans? First, they eat a huge amount of soy, nearly 100 grams per day. This is more than twice the amount of soy protein consumed by mainland Japanese and 25 times more soy than consumed by Americans. At the same time, they limit their calorie intake, consuming nearly 30 percent fewer calories than the Japanese. How do they decrease calorie intake while simultaneously increasing soy intake? By cutting down on rice while stocking up on vegetables, thus reducing the amount of carbohydrates consumed. Essentially, they are following an eating plan that is very similar to the Zone, particularly the Soy Zone.

As I explain in greater detail in Chapter 9, there are two main reasons why the Okinawan diet will improve longevity. First, soy protein decreases insulin levels, to an even greater degree than animal protein. Second, the restricted calorie intake lowers the levels of free radicals in your body, the damaging elements that can speed aging. Both of these anti-aging benefits can also be obtained by following a Zone diet rich in soy protein. You will learn all about the anti-aging process in Chapter 9, but for now just remember to add more soy to your diet, using protein powder, tofu, tempeh, soy hot dogs, soy sausages, or soy hamburgers.

This soy recommendation applies even if you are not a vegetarian, since many of the health and hormonal benefits of soy cannot be obtained as effectively from animal protein. Likewise, if you have already stopped eating meat, consuming more soy is particularly crucial because many vegetarian diets are too high in pasta, bread, and rice and too low in protein. You may have turned to a vegetarian diet to achieve better health, only to find that your health has begun to decline. Perhaps you have gained weight, or have been plagued by persistent colds and fatigue. These are all signs that you are out of the Zone, and have been eating too many high-density carbs and not enough protein. Soy protein can get you into the Zone, and keep you there forever. Not only will you gain all the advantages of the Zone, you'll also reap the health rewards that soy can provide.

Just to show how easy this is, I have listed some of the Vegetarian Zone meals from *The Soy Zone*.

Asparagus Frittata

1 Breakfast or Dinner Entrée

Ingredients
4 ounces firm tofu, cubed
1 whole egg
2 egg whites
¼ teaspoon dried basil
¼ teaspoon ground black pepper
¼ teaspoon sea salt
½ cup unsweetened tomato sauce
1 small onion, thinly sliced
1 bunch asparagus (about 8–10 stalks)
1 large red or yellow bell pepper, cut into ¼-inch strips
1⅓ teaspoons olive oil
pinch of salt

Instructions
1 Preheat oven to 400°.
2. In a medium bowl, mash tofu with a fork. Add egg, egg whites, basil, black pepper, and salt. Whisk mixture with fork and set aside.
3. Pour tomato sauce into small saucepan and gently warm over low heat.
4. Meanwhile, fill a large pot with lid with ½ inch water. Set steamer basket into pot and layer onions, asparagus, and bell pepper into steamer. Cover pot and bring to boil over high heat.

Reduce to medium heat and steam vegetables 5 to 6 minutes, or until just tender. If you don't have a steamer, boil the vegetables till tender, about 3 minutes. Transfer to plate.

5: In a medium oven-proof skillet, heat oil over medium-high flame until oil sizzles. Pour in egg/tofu mixture all at once and reduce heat to medium-low. Spread egg/tofu mixture evenly across pan to cook.

6: Before mixture has completely set, evenly distribute steamed vegetables over eggs. Transfer skillet to oven and cook for about 5 minutes, or until egg/tofu mixture completely sets and vegetables are hot. Add a pinch of salt and serve with tomato sauce.

Greek Salad With Garlic-Oregano Dressing

1 Lunch or Dinner Entrée

Ingredients

5 cups loosely packed romaine lettuce, washed, patted dry, and torn into small pieces

1 cup canned artichoke hearts, drained and cut into bite-size pieces

2 medium tomatoes, cut into wedges

1 small red onion, thinly sliced

¼ cup canned garbanzo beans, drained and rinsed

2 ounces feta cheese, crumbled

6 ounces extra-firm tofu, cut into ½-inch cubes

1⅓ teaspoons extra-virgin olive oil

1 tablespoon red wine vinegar

2 tablespoons vegetable stock or water

1 small garlic clove, minced

¼ teaspoon dried oregano, crumbled

¼ teaspoon freshly ground black pepper

Instructions

1: Arrange lettuce on large dinner plate. Top with artichoke hearts, tomatoes, onions, garbanzo beans, feta cheese, and tofu.

2: In a small bowl, mix together olive oil, red wine vinegar, vegetable stock or water, garlic, oregano, and black pepper. Pour over salad and toss to evenly distribute dressing. Serve.

Variation: If you have it on hand, try using cold baked or cold grilled tofu in this recipe. Many health food stores now carry pre-baked or pregrilled tofu in the refrigerator section.

Easy Barbecue Tempeh and Vegetables

1 Dinner Entrée

Ingredients
1⅓ teaspoons olive oil
½ small onion, diced
2 medium stalks celery, diced
1 clove garlic, pressed
1 red or green bell pepper, diced
4 ounces tempeh, cubed
⅓ cup textured vegetable protein (such as Morningstar Farms Burger Style Recipe Crumbles)
½ to ¾ cup vegetable broth
1 teaspoon prepared mustard
1 teaspoon apple cider vinegar
2 tablespoons prepared barbecue sauce

Instructions

1: Heat oil in large skillet and sauté onions and celery over medium-high heat until onions are translucent and slightly browned.
2: Add garlic, bell pepper, tempeh, and textured vegetable protein and sauté 3 to 5 minutes longer. If the mixture starts sticking to skillet, add 2 to 3 tablespoons vegetable broth.
3: Add vegetable broth, mustard, vinegar, and barbecue sauce. Simmer covered about 20 minutes, until tempeh is infused with flavor.

Very Berry Smoothie

4 Snack Portions or 1 Breakfast Entrée

Ingredients
⅓ cup unsweetened pineapple juice
1⅓ ounces unflavored soy protein powder (portion containing
    28 grams protein)
½ teaspoon pure vanilla extract
⅛ teaspoon ground nutmeg
1 cup frozen, unsweetened blueberries
1 heaping cup frozen, unsweetened strawberries
1⅓ teaspoons olive oil or almond oil

Instructions

1: Place juice and protein powder in blender container. Cover and blend until smooth.
2: Add vanilla, nutmeg, blueberries, strawberries, and oil. Blend until smooth, scraping down sides of blender if necessary.

Variation: For a thicker, icier smoothie, add 4 or 5 ice cubes.

9

THE ANTI-AGING ZONE: LIVING LONGER AND LIVING BETTER

et's face it: We all want to stay young forever. We do everything in our power to reverse signs of aging, from buying fancy face creams that are "age-defying" to expensive cosmetic surgery like facelifts. We're all looking for that quick fix that can turn back the clock—no matter what the cost.

Now I'm going to give you a proposal. Let's say you can reverse the aging process simply by changing your lifestyle. You'll look younger, have the strength and stamina that you had 20 years earlier, and prevent those diseases that are telltale signs of age: heart disease, osteoporosis, cancer. Interested?

I thought you would be. In fact, I wrote an entire book called *The Anti-Aging Zone* that details how the Zone Diet works hand in hand with various lifestyle factors to reverse the aging process. The centerpiece of this plan is what I call the Anti-Aging Zone Lifestyle Pyramid. By employing the strategies outlined at each level of the pyramid, you'll be able to conquer what I call the four pillars of aging: excess insulin, excess free radicals, excess cortisol, and excess blood sugar. Each of these pillars acts in a different way to corrupt your hormonal communication system and accelerate aging.

My point is that the aging process can be reversed if you are willing to incorporate some basic lifestyle strategies into your daily activities that will fine-tune your hormonal systems. The key strategies include calorie restriction using the Zone Diet, moderate exercise, and stress reduction through meditation. Unfortunately, exercise and meditation are not equal to the Zone Diet in terms of their ability to reverse aging: following the Zone Diet is by far the most important step in your anti-aging efforts. I've ranked these strategies in order of importance and come up with the Lifestyle Pyramid that you see below.

Anti-Aging Zone Lifestyle Pyramid

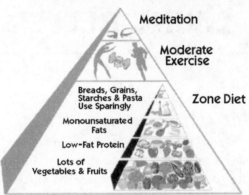

The base of the pyramid, which takes up the largest block of space, contains the most important component of the anti-aging lifestyle: a calorie-restricted diet, in particular the Zone Diet. Calorie restriction is the only scientifically proven method to reverse aging. The verdict is definitely in that it works. As I mentioned earlier, the Zone Diet naturally restricts your calories by limiting your intake of high-density carbohydrates. It provides far greater hormonal benefits than any other calorie-restricted diet and doesn't leave you feeling hungry and deprived, like diets based primarily on grains and other starches. Without following the Zone Diet, you simply won't be able to achieve the maximum benefits of age reversal.

The next step of the Zone Anti-Aging Lifestyle Pyramid is moderate exercise. Although the question of whether intensive exercise extends your lifespan remains unanswered, a lack of exercise, without a doubt, increases the aging process. With exercise, you need to strike the right balance. Intense levels of exercise put stress on the body by increasing the formation of free radicals and increasing levels of the stress hormone cortisol—both of which can speed aging. You want to aim for moderate but consistent exercise. You also need to keep in mind that even the best exercise program can be obliterated by the wrong diet.

At the top of the Lifestyle Pyramid, you'll find stress reduction, particularly through meditation. Meditation can help reverse the damage caused by stress by lowering levels of stress hormones, especially cortisol. Unfortunately, the jury is still out over whether meditation can actually increase your longevity. In theory, though, meditation should delay aging in the brain by protecting it against the ravages caused by excess production of cortisol. Just like exercise, meditation can't do the anti-aging job alone. You need to combine it with a hormonally correct diet like the Zone.

If you combine all three components of the Lifestyle Pyramid, you'll start disassociating your biological age (i.e., how your body functions and feels) from your chronological age (the number of candles on the cake). That means you may be 60, but look and perform like a 40-year-old, or be a 40-year-old and look and perform like a 20-year-old. The Zone Anti-Aging Lifestyle Pyramid can actually turn back your physiological age by 20 years! The key is to make these lifestyle changes permanent. Depending on how you choose to live your life, you are either speeding or reversing the aging process each day. At the end of each day (or even at the end of every meal), you should ask yourself: "Did I take steps to lengthen my life span or to shorten it?" Even if you're disappointed by your answer, remember that tomorrow you'll have another chance to reverse your physiological age.

How the Zone Reverses Aging

I believe that the Zone Diet is the single most important thing you can do to reverse aging for this reason: it reduces all four pillars of aging simultaneously. Following the Zone Diet, you'll restrict your calorie intake, which will reduce the formation of tissue-damaging free radicals. At the same time, you'll also reduce excess blood glucose because you are not consuming excess amounts of carbohydrates. By the same token, you'll reduce excess insulin, which is triggered by excess carbohydrate consumption. Last, you'll reduce the likelihood of excess cortisol production to maintain blood glucose levels, since at every meal you'll eat adequate levels of low-fat protein, which stimulates the secretion of glucagon (the hormone that restores blood glucose levels).

You don't need any special adaptations to the Zone Diet to maximize its age-reversing benefits. Simply follow the concepts that I outlined in the previous chapters, and you'll be taking the most important step you can take to reverse aging.

The next level of the Anti-Aging Zone Lifestyle Pyramid is moderate exercise. With the exercise component, you want to have a cross-training program that affects as many hormonal systems as possible. To reduce insulin, you should plan to do 30 minutes of aerobic exercise every day: brisk walking is one of your best exercise choices, but you can also play volleyball, run, swim, or take a step class. Try several types of exercise and find out what you really enjoy. In addition, you want to spend 5 to 10 minutes a day on a strength-training program.

Strength training is not thought of fondly by most people, but it is the only form of exercise that will build and maintain the muscle mass necessary for maximal functioning in the future. For upper-body strength, the best exercise is push-ups. The word *push-up* conveys dread in most individuals. Therefore, if you are not physically fit, start your daily strength exercise with push-aways from a wall. Stand two to three feet from a wall and extend your hands in a direct line from your shoulders until they reach the wall. Make sure the placement of the hands is low enough on the wall so that when you lower yourself your shoulders will be just above your hands. Lower your body toward the wall, and then push away to return to the original position. Do three sets of 10 to 15 repetitions with a one-minute rest in between sets.

If you can do this easily, then graduate to counter push-backs. Stand two to three feet from a countertop (again positioning your hands in a direct line from the shoulder) and extend your hands to reach the top of the counter. (When lowering yourself to the counter, your shoulders should be directly over your hands). Lower your body to the counter, and then push back to the original position. As you originally did with the push-aways from the wall, do three sets of countertop push-backs each with 10 to 15 repetitions.

Once these are mastered, then move to the knee push-up. Here you are on the floor with your knees bent and your arms extended to the floor (again in a direct line from your shoulder). Lower yourself until your chest (not your stomach) touches the floor, and then raise yourself back up to the original position. Once you have mastered this exercise for 10 to 15 repetitions in three sets, then you are ready to graduate to the dreaded push-up in which only your toes are touching the ground and your arms are totally extended (again so the hands and shoulders are in a direct line). Lower yourself to the floor until your chest reaches it, and then return to the original position. Once you can achieve 10 to 15 repetitions for three sets, then you have two additional options. One is to simply do more repetitions of push-ups in each set. The other is to raise your feet off the floor (like on a chair) and then do your push-ups. Of the two, the first (more repetitions) is easier and probably safer. Don't be disappointed if you have to start with the wall push-aways due to lack of current upper-body strength. It just means you have greater potential for improvement.

The best exercise for developing lower-body strength is the squat. In earlier days it was known as a deep knee bend. Just like the push-up, you start this exercise slowly, depending on your initial fitness level. As a start, just stand facing forward in front of a chair that has arms. Place your hands on the arms of the chair, and then slowly lower yourself to the seat of the chair. Still using the arms of the chair for support, raise yourself back up to a standing position. Do three sets of 10 to 15 repetitions with a one-minute rest between each set.

The next step is to do the same exercise, but without using the arms of the chair for support (however, the arms are always there to be used for support if needed, like a safety net). Again, your goal is to achieve 10 to 15 repetitions in three sets.

Graduating to the next level means using a chair with no arms. With your arms crossed over your chest, you do your squat. As you did with the push-ups, simply increase your repetitions until you reach 15 repetitions per set.

This strength-training program will take less than 10 minutes per day. Regardless of your fitness level, these exercises for upper- and lower-body strength should be done every day. Since they don't require any equipment, they can be done at home or on the road.

There is simply no excuse not to make them part of your Anti-Aging Zone Lifestyle.

These exercises (brisk walking and simple strength-training exercises) should be the core of your moderate exercise program. But this doesn't mean that more exercises can't be added. For more aerobic intensity, think about walking on hilly terrain as opposed to a flat landscape. When you travel, this might mean walking up and down the stairs of your hotel. Alternatively, you may want to invest in a home exercise machine like a rower, a stationary bicycle, or a treadmill to increase the intensity of the workout, or decrease the time spent exercising aerobically so that you get your 300 calories of daily energy expenditure. This will provide 2,000 calories per week of exercise, which provides maximum longevity benefits. For additional anaerobic training, you might want to get a set of adjustable dumbbells because they are easily stored and provide maximum flexibility in the number of weight-training exercises you can do. If you do any additional strength training, never do more than 45 minutes of strength training because beyond that point, cortisol levels begin to rise. Extended strength training beyond this time frame in a single session will start to accelerate the aging process.

Monitoring Your Progress

Since maintaining strength will be one of your most important components of functionality, you need to have some indication of how you are progressing on this component of your Anti-Aging Zone Lifestyle. Here's how you can measure your strength at home.

For determining your upper-body strength, males will do standard push-ups and females will do knee push-ups. Always make sure that your back is not sagging (just pull your abdominals in) and that you are touching the floor with your chest and not your chin. In other words, the number you can do is based on maintaining perfect form. Remember, no one is watching you, so you want to get a true test of your current upper-body strength.

Push-ups: Men

AGE:	20–29	30–39	40–49	50–59	60
EXCELLENT	55	45	40	35	30
GOOD	45–54	35–44	30–39	25–34	20–29
AVERAGE	35–44	25–34	20–29	15–24	10–19
FAIR	20–34	15–24	12–19	8–14	5–9
LOW	0–19	0–14	0–11	0–7	0–4

Knee Push-ups: Women

AGE:	20–29	30–39	40–49	50–59	60
EXCELLENT	49	40	35	30	20
GOOD	34–48	25–39	20–34	15–29	5–19
AVERAGE	17–33	12–24	8–19	6–14	3–4
FAIR	6–16	4–11	3–7	2–5	1–2
LOW	0–5	0–3	0–2	0–1	0

Don't be dismayed if you have a low score. Most Americans will. In fact, the average male teenager can't do 10 push-ups. But with consistent exercise, your upper-body strength will increase.

Lower-body strength is measured by the number of times you can do a squat with weights. Use a chair of standard height (approximately 18–20 inches) without arms. Males should hold 15-pound dumbbells in each hand (a total of 30 pounds), and females should hold 5-pound dumbbells in each hand (a total of 10 pounds). Keeping your legs open as wide as your hips, do a standard squat until you touch the seat of the chair and then return to your starting position. Do as many standard squats as you can while maintaining good form. Then check out how you rate in lower-body strength.

30-Pound Squats: Men

AGE:	20–29	30–39	40–49	50–59	60
EXCELLENT	55	45	40	35	30
GOOD	45–54	35–44	30–39	25–34	20–29
AVERAGE	35–44	25–34	20–29	15–24	10–19
FAIR	20–34	15–24	12–19	8–14	5–9
LOW	0–19	0–14	0–11	0–7	0–4

10-Pound Squats: Women

AGE:	20–29	30–39	40–49	50–59	60
EXCELLENT	49	40	35	30	20
GOOD	34–48	25–39	20–34	15–29	5–19
AVERAGE	17–33	12–24	8–19	6–14	3–4
FAIR	6–16	4–11	3–7	2–5	1–2
LOW	0–5	0–3	0–2	0–1	0

Finally, your cross-training program should include flexibility exercises. In addition to five minutes of stretching to warm up and cool down before and after more intensive exercises, you should plan to do at least 20 minutes every other day of continuous stretching. It doesn't matter if it's basic sports stretching or yoga; both are great.

So here is your basic Anti-Aging Zone exercise program:

1. 30 minutes of brisk walking every day.
2. 5 to 10 minutes of basic strength-building exercises (push-ups and squats) every day.

So far, not too hard. Try to do this every day, but if you do these basic exercises at least five days a week, you will be making progress in your anti-aging program. Then, if you want to add to this basic program, consider the following:

1. Replace your daily brisk walk with a slightly higher-intensity aerobic exercise (rowing, bicycling, or walking on a treadmill where you can increase the difficulty) until you have burned 300–400 calories. If the machine doesn't have a calorie counter, this would be about 30 minutes of exercise.
2. Do no more than 45 minutes of strength training with dumbbells (or free weights and exercise machines) three days per week.
3. Do 20 minutes of flexibility exercises on the days that you don't do any strength training.

The moderate exercise component of the Zone Anti-Aging Lifestyle Pyramid will reduce excess insulin and excess blood sugar, two of the four pillars of aging, without increasing cortisol or free radicals. Not quite as good as reducing all four pillars of aging as with the Zone Diet, but by increasing strength and aerobic fitness, you will increase your functionality in later life.

The final component of the Zone Anti-Aging Lifestyle Pyramid is meditation, because it can lower at least one pillar of aging: excess cortisol production, which is important for promoting brain longevity.

Meditation is not simply sitting back and thinking good thoughts or daydreaming. It is a very precise way to control cortisol. Meditation for the specific physiological purpose of cortisol reduction is key to your brain longevity program. This is not to say that the use of meditation to achieve spiritual goals is not a higher purpose, but that requires a far greater commitment. Here we are simply looking at meditation as another anti-aging tool. This is a very Western (i.e., goal-oriented) approach. In essence, it is practical meditation.

PRACTICAL MEDITATION

Practical meditation is not some purely mystical technique known only to a few gurus. Practical meditation is a series of defined actions. There appear to be common themes that run throughout recorded history on how to meditate. There is usually a constant chanting of a word or phrase or a focus on a physiological action (such as breathing), always returning to that focus on a word, phrase, or physiological function when your thoughts begin to wander (i.e., daydreaming). In essence, you are trying to clear the decks mentally.

Here is a thumbnail sketch of practical meditation: Find a quiet place with a comfortable chair. Close your eyes and repeat a word (the word *one* is a good choice) or phrase continually. At the same time, focus on your breathing. Try to always expand your stomach when you inhale. By focusing on the word or phrase and your breathing, you are trying to keep random thoughts from coming into your consciousness. If such random thoughts do appear, simply refocus your attention on the word and your breathing until they pass. Do this for 20 minutes a day, and there you have it, practical meditation.

Meditation (even practical meditation) takes practice (just like the Zone Diet and exercise), but with increasing skill, significant physiological changes related to reduction of cortisol levels can be achieved. These include the reduction of blood pressure and heart rate, and improvement in immune function.

Do practical meditation for 20 minutes a day, and you have a proven drug to reduce cortisol levels. It's a simple technique that helps alter hormonal response and in the process improves brain longevity.

The same three "drugs"—the Zone Diet, moderate exercise, and practical meditation—that can alter the pillars of aging for your body can also alter the hormonal environment in which the brain must function. Your ability to use these "drugs" correctly will determine how well you play the longevity game. Look around you, and see how you compare to your peers. Do you look younger? Are you in better shape? Do you have more energy? Are you more mentally alert? If so, you are younger than your years. If not, you're older. Aging is more than a state of mind; it requires constant application of the Anti-Aging Zone Lifestyle Pyramid. If you decide to throw in the towel and let your good lifestyle habits slide, you'll find yourself feeling older and weaker. If you choose to take charge and live a healthy life in the Zone, you'll stay strong and young for the rest of your life. The choice is up to you.

10

ZONE SUPPLEMENTS

So by following the Zone, engaging in moderate daily exercise, and practicing meditation, you have a great battle plan for a longer and better life. But what about all the vitamins and minerals that are supposed to reverse aging? Actually, it's macronutrients (protein, carbohydrate, and fat) that are your passport to the Zone, not micronutrient (vitamins and minerals) supplements. Are supplements important for the Zone? A few are, but never let the tail wag the dog. Supplements can enhance your experience in the Zone, but supplements will never get you into the Zone on their own.

What about vitamins and minerals? Isn't our food more deficient in these essential micronutrients than it was 50 years ago? The answer is yes. Why? Fifty years ago, most of the fruits and vegetables came from your backyard or just outside town at the nearby farm. Now they come from all over the world and can be stored for months after being harvested. Vitamins are incredibly sensitive to heat, light, and storage time. Minerals are more stable, but they are very sensitive to processing and cooking technologies. The first casualties in the war for cheap food will always be the vitamin and mineral content of that food. So should you spend a good chunk of your food bill down at the local health food store buying expensive vitamin and mineral supplements? No, but you can use certain supplements wisely to get the most out of the Zone Diet.

Not all vitamins and minerals are of equal importance. I list them below in terms of their importance.

ESSENTIAL SUPPLEMENTS

These are purified fish oils and Vitamin E. Here the research is overpowering, and their cost is relatively inexpensive in comparison to the enhanced health benefits they provide.

Fish Oil

Let's talk about fish oil first, since your grandmother probably used it in the form of cod liver oil. Cod liver oil is rich in Vitamin A and Vitamin D, and was used two generations ago to prevent a disease called rickets. Even though it was (and probably still is) one of the most disgusting foods known to man, its daily consumption was a given.

It turns out that the real reason that cod liver oil was so beneficial was not because of the vitamins it contained, but because of its high levels of the long-chain omega-3 fatty acids called eicospentaenoic acid (EPA) and docosahexaenoic acid (DHA). EPA turns out to be a key factor for controlling insulin levels, and DHA is needed to maintain and rebuild your brain. So even though your grandmother was forcing your parents to eat cod liver oil for the wrong biochemical reasons, she was doing an excellent job of controlling insulin and improving brain longevity. In fact, as I explain in *The Soy Zone*, DHA was the transformational factor that made modern man the master of the planet. Without adequate levels of DHA, your brain-power drops significantly. Equally important, many neurological conditions such as depression, multiple sclerosis, and attention deficit disorders are linked to low levels of DHA in the diet, and often supplementation with fish oils rich in DHA can show dramatic changes within a few weeks.

The need for these long-chain omega-3 fatty acids is only now being realized. Fifty percent of the weight of the brain is composed of fat. And one-third of the brain's mass is composed of long-chain omega-3 fats, like DHA. No other organ in the body has such a concentration of DHA. The greatest growth spurt for the brain occurs during the first two years of life, which is why human breast milk is so rich in DHA. Just how important are these omega-3 fats found in breast milk? One English study indicated that breast-fed children scored nearly 10 points higher on IQ tests compared to children who were formula-fed.

Just as DHA is important for the brain, EPA is also incredibly beneficial in reducing heart disease, cancer, arthritis, and other chronic disease conditions in humans. Why? Because of its effect on a group of hormones called eicosanoids. Why eicosanoids are so important is described in detail in *The Zone* and *The Anti-Aging Zone*, but simply stated, if you want to decrease the likelihood of developing most chronic diseases, then adequate intake of EPA from fish oils is key.

My prescription for fish oil: Even if you are eating two to three servings of fish per week, I still recommend taking a fish oil supplement of about 5 grams per day. That's about one teaspoon of fish oil. Fortunately, today's fish oils are nearly tasteless and can be taken in capsule form.

Vitamin E

The other essential vitamin supplement for the Zone Diet is Vitamin E. It is simply impossible to obtain adequate levels of Vitamin E through diet alone. As with fish oil, the data are compelling that increased supplementation with Vitamin E will have a dramatic clinical effect on diseases ranging from heart disease to Alzheimer's and immune system disorders. The primary benefit of Vitamin E is the destruction of fat-soluble free radicals.

My prescription for Vitamin E: I recommend taking a minimum of 100 I.U. per day, with 400 I.U. as a reasonable upper limit for adults and 50 to 100 I.U. a reasonable upper limit for children (because of their lower body weight).

IMPORTANT SUPPLEMENTS

If fish oils and Vitamin E are essential supplements for the Zone Diet (and any other diet for that matter), then there is a second tier of vitamins and minerals that I consider very important for anyone interested in their health. This tier of supplements includes Vitamin C and the mineral magnesium.

Vitamin C

Vitamin C is an anti-oxidant that reduces excess water-soluble free radicals (one of the pillars of aging). Vitamin C acts like a shuttle to get rid of all the nasty fat-soluble oxidation products that are constantly being formed in your body. And if you don't have enough Vitamin C, these oxidation products pile up and get stored in your fat cells, where they can cause trouble.

Fortunately, Vitamin C is plentiful, especially when following the Zone Diet. Unlike Vitamin E and purified fish oils, where supplementation is a must, fruits and vegetables tend to be rich in Vitamin C. The best sources of Vitamin C in fruits are kiwis, oranges, and strawberries. Vegetables such as red peppers, broccoli, spinach, and mustard greens are also rich in Vitamin C.

My prescription for Vitamin C: Although megadoses of Vitamin C are often touted, the best research indicates that a reasonable level for Vitamin C supplementation is in the range of 250 to 500 mg per day. Because Vitamin C is so inexpensive, supplementation of this vitamin is a good recommendation for everyone.

Magnesium

The one mineral supplement I highly recommend is magnesium. No mineral is as important as magnesium in the Zone. It's the critical mineral cofactor for the enzymes involved in the production of eicosanoids. In addition, it is a cofactor for more than 350 other enzymes. The latest research shows that adequate magnesium is critical for cardiovascular patients, which only makes it reasonable to assume that it is useful for the rest of us, especially since dietary surveys indicate that nearly 75 percent of Americans are deficient in this key mineral. Magnesium is found in every green vegetable, such as spinach and broccoli. However, the richest naturally occurring sources of magnesium are nuts. Other sources that are relatively rich in magnesium are leafy green vegetables, and seafoods like shrimp and crab. These foods are also among the primary foods used in the Zone Diet. Also not surprising is that the foods that are poor in magnesium are starches, breads, and pasta, the new staples of the American diet. No wonder Americans are magnesium-deficient.

My prescription for magnesium: Store-bought magnesium supplements are difficult to take because magnesium tastes terrible and is poorly absorbed by the body. So go the natural route first. Eat lots of nuts (especially those rich in monounsaturated fat, like almonds and cashews), and the other foods rich in magnesium. If you insist on taking store-bought supplements, the cheapest are capsules of magnesium oxide. Capsules containing the chelated magnesium (for better absorption) actually have less magnesium per capsule and are more expensive. Regardless of the dosage form, try to take 300 to 400 mg of supplemental magnesium per day.

CHEAP INSURANCE POLICIES

I think of the third-tier supplements as cheap insurance policies. Although their benefits to an individual on the Zone Diet are limited compared to the benefits of the supplements recommended above, these supplements represent a very inexpensive way to create peace of mind.

Beta-carotene

The first of these third-tier supplements is beta-carotene. No supplement in the world causes more confusion than beta-carotene. Scientists always want to search for a magic bullet that can be put into a capsule and sold as the essence of health. For many years beta-carotene seemed to be such a magic bullet. After all, there were many studies showing that higher blood levels of beta-carotene were associated with lower risks of heart disease and cancer. The obvious conclusion was that beta-carotene was the key factor for preventing both diseases, but in this case the scientists were looking at the tree instead of the forest.

No one thought for a minute that the reason there was a lot of beta-carotene in the bloodstream of healthy people was that these people were eating a lot of fruit! After all, if you are eating a lot of fruit, it is unlikely that you are eating a lot of high-density carbohydrates, such as starches and pasta. It's now clear that beta-carotene didn't have the mystical properties that researchers first thought; in fact, it's just as possible that all the healthy fruit eaters had lower rates of heart disease and cancer because they were keeping insulin levels low by not eating as many high-density carbohydrates.

Another important fact to remember about beta-carotene is that it must be taken with Vitamin C. Beta-carotene is a great anti-oxidant for fat-soluble free radicals (just like Vitamin E). This simply means it picks up free radicals and stabilizes them before they can do some real damage. But unless removed from the body, a stabi-lized free radical is still trouble looking to strike. To get these free radicals out of your system, you need adequate levels of water-soluble anti-oxidants (like Vitamin C) to take the free radicals from beta-carotene and transport them to the liver, where they can be excreted. And that was the problem with the beta-carotene studies: you have to add extra Vitamin C to transport the beta-carotene-stabilized free radicals to the liver for their final detoxification.

Does this mean that beta-carotene is somehow dangerous or a supplement you should avoid? Of course not, and in fact it has great utility as long as the other part of the equation (Vitamin C) is pres-ent at adequate levels. This is why Vitamin C is very important as a Zone supplement, and beta-carotene is less important.

My prescription for beta-carotene: I usually recommend 5,000 I.U. of beta-carotene as a supplement. But before you go out and buy extra beta-carotene supplements, try getting it from fruits and from vegetables like red peppers and spinach. And while carrots contain beta-carotene, unfortunately they enter the bloodstream very rapidly, thus raising insulin levels, which can be worse for your health than the benefit gained by the increase in beta-carotene.

Other supplements that I place into this third tier are Vitamins B3 (niacin) and B6 (pyridoxine), which are critical for the produc-tion of eicosanoids.

Niacin

Lack of niacin was discovered as the cause of pellagra. It became a widespread epidemic in this country at the turn of the century when poorer populations subsisted on white flour, white rice, and sugar, products all devoid of niacin. (Not surprisingly, these foods have become the staples of our country but now in the form of pasta, bagels, and rice cakes). Unlike most vitamins, niacin can be produced in the body through the conversion of the amino acid tryptophan into niacin. However, the process is not very efficient, but it does mean that if you are eating adequate levels of protein, you will probably avert an outright deficiency of niacin. The best source of niacin remains food, and particularly foods that are integral to the Zone Diet, including lean meat, poultry, fish, eggs, cheese, and milk. While whole grains are another good source, I don't recommend them because their higher carbohydrate densities will increase insulin levels, thus outweighing any benefit of increased niacin.

My prescription for niacin: If you are going to supplement with niacin, then 20 mg per day is a good dose.

Pyridoxine (Vitamin B6)

As with niacin, increased food processing has reduced the amount of Vitamin B6 in our food. This vitamin is a vital co-factor for making eicosanoids, so its presence is important.

My prescription for pyridoxine: I would recommend 5 to 10 mg per day. These amounts of B6 vitamin can also be found in any decent vitamin pill.

Folic Acid

Folic acid is another vitamin that has received research attention because of its ability to reduce both neural tube defects in children and levels of homocysteine, a risk factor for heart disease. The name folic acid comes from the Latin word for leaf because that is exactly where you find this vitamin—in leafy green vegetables.

My prescription for folic acid: Although the RDA for this vitamin is 200 micrograms per day, the most recent research (especially on heart disease) indicates that it makes sense to take at least 500 to 1,000 micrograms per day. It turns out that folic acid also works with Vitamins B3 and B6 to reduce the levels of homocysteine, another example of vitamin synergy (like Vitamin C and Vitamin E) in the body.

In this same tier of useful supplements are the minerals calcium, zinc, selenium, and chromium.

Calcium

You have been told that calcium is necessary for strong bones, since 99 percent of the calcium in your body is in your bones. But it's also needed to control muscle contraction and nerve conduction. Dairy products, including cheese, are without a doubt the best sources of calcium. Our national fat phobia has made most dairy products *persona non grata*, forcing many women to go out and get calcium supplements. But dairy products aren't the only sources of calcium because broccoli, cauliflower, green leafy vegetables, and calcium-precipitated tofu also provide this important mineral.

My prescription for calcium: I recommend 500 to 1,000 mg of calcium per day. Much of this can be obtained from low-fat dairy products.

Zinc

Another important mineral to consider is zinc. Zinc plays a critical role in the proper functioning of your immune system and, not surprisingly, in the production of eicosanoids. As you might expect, good sources of zinc are the building blocks of the Zone Diet, including chicken, beef, fish, oatmeal, and nuts.

My prescription for zinc: If you are going to supplement with zinc, then 15 mg per day should be sufficient. As with Vitamins B3 and B6, you will probably find this amount of zinc in a typical vitamin/mineral supplement.

Selenium

Another important mineral is selenium, which is an essential component of the enzyme known as glutathione peroxidase, which reduces excess free radicals. This is why selenium supplementation is useful in cancer treatment and prevention. Food sources higher on the food chain tend to be rich in selenium. These include seafood and beef. Nuts are also rich in selenium.

My prescription for selenium: The dose I advise for this supplement is 200 micrograms per day, and L-selenomethionine is your best store-bought choice for maximum selenium absorption.

Chromium

Chromium is part of a biochemical complex known as glucose tolerance factor. This complex makes insulin more effective in driving blood glucose into cells for utilization. Therefore, the more chromium you have, the less insulin you need to make. This is why chromium is called a potentiator of insulin action. Unfortunately, many supplement manufacturers have touted chromium as the only nutrient required to lose fat or gain muscle mass. Nothing can be further from the truth. Your diet will have a far greater effect on insulin than any supplement.

My prescription for chromium: If you choose to supplement your diet with chromium, I suggest taking approximately 200 micrograms per day.

EXOTIC AND NOT-SO-CHEAP SUPPLEMENTS

This last group of vitamins is interesting, but only if you have money to spare. It includes lycopene, leutin, CoQ10, and oligoproanthocyanidins. All are exotic anti-oxidants. Two of the most interesting are the carotenoids lycopene and leutin.

Lycopene and Lutein

Lycopene has been associated with a decrease in prostate cancer and is found primarily in foods with red pigments, such as tomato and watermelon. Lutein is associated with a decrease in macular degeneration (which causes an ever-decreasing field of vision in the eye and leads to blindness). Where do you find lutein? In green leafy vegetables and red peppers.

My recommendations for lycopene and leutin: If you want to supplement your diet with these very expensive anti-oxidants, try 3 to 5 mg per day.

CoQ10

This is really not a vitamin, since the body can synthesize it, but the synthesis is usually very inefficient. CoQ10 functions like a souped-up Vitamin E and appears to be the last line of defense for preventing the oxidation of low-density lipoproteins (LDL), which appear to be a major factor in the development of atherosclerosis. There is also evidence of its benefit in the treatment of congestive heart failure.

My prescription for CoQ10: I recommend 30 mg per day.

Oligoproanthocyanidins (OPC)

These anti-oxidants are also known as polyphenolics. They are found in grapes and are part of the bioflavanoid family, which works together with Vitamin C. Since bioflavanoids have some solubility in both fats and water, they make a good shuttle system to help move stabilized free radicals from fat-soluble anti-oxidants, such as Vitamin E and beta-carotene, to water-soluble anti-oxidants, such as Vitamin C. The end result is that excess free radicals can be detoxified by the liver more rapidly.

My prescription for OPC: I would suggest 5 to 10 mg per day.

SUPPLEMENTS FOR VEGETARIANS

Although my recommendations are always the same for vegetarians, there are two special additions.

DHA from Algae

The only way that vegetarians can get adequate levels of the long-chain omega-3 fatty acid DHA, which is critical for brain function, is with supplementation. DHA can now be isolated from algae. The body will retroconvert some of this supplemented DHA into EPA. A far less efficient way is to consume large amounts of flaxseed oil. Even though flaxseed oil contains short-chain omega-3 fatty acids, their conversion into long-chain omega-3 fatty acids is very inefficient.

My prescription for algae-based DHA: 3 to 5 grams of algae oil (containing at least 1 gram of DHA total).

Vitamin B12

The one other supplement for vegetarians is Vitamin B12, since it is only found in animal protein sources.

My prescription for Vitamin B12: Because of the poor absorption of Vitamin B12, I would recommend taking 50 micrograms per day.

Summary of Recommendations

Type	Daily Amount
Essential	
Fish oil	5 grams
Vitamin E	100–400 I.U.
Important	
Vitamin C	250–500 mg
Magnesium	300–400 mg
Cheap Insurance	
Beta-carotene	5,000 I.U.
Vitamin B3 (niacin)	20 mg
Vitamin B6 (pyridoxine)	5–10 mg
Folic acid	500–1,000 ug
Calcium	500–1,000 mg
Zinc	15 mg
Selenium	200 ug
Chromium	200 ug
Exotic and Not-So-Cheap Insurance	
Lycopene	3–5 mg
Lutein	3–5 mg
CoQ10	30 mg
OPC	5–10 mg
Supplements for Vegetarians	
Algae oil containing DHA	3–5 grams
Vitamin B12	50 ug

11

FINE-TUNING THE ZONE

This will help you further master the Zone. If you are doing well using the eye-and-palm method, then you don't have to read this chapter carefully. However, the information contained in this chapter will enable you to fine-tune the Zone to your unique biochemistry.

The Zone is not a diet in the traditional sense. Diets can be thought of as short-term periods of deprivation and hunger to lose excess weight, only to return to your old eating habits, which originally caused the weight gain in the first place. The Zone Diet is a lifelong food management program based on balance and moderation for better insulin control. Think of the Zone as a hormonal checkbook. Like your regular checkbook, you don't have to balance it to the penny to make it work. You only want to assure yourself that there is enough money in the account so that the next check you write doesn't bounce. The Zone is similar. You want the best possible balance of protein, carbohydrate, and fat at each meal to achieve the right hormonal action, but you don't have to balance your meal to the exact gram each and every time.

YOUR HORMONAL CARBURETOR

The Zone Diet can be viewed as the constant balancing of protein to carbohydrate at every meal and snack to get the best hormonal output. This is similar in concept to balancing the gas and air in your car engine to get the best mileage. There is no one exact ratio for the optimal balance because of the genetic diversity of individuals. However, the balance of protein to carbohydrate can be described in terms of a bell curve, as shown below.

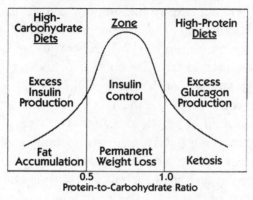

Entering the Zone Depends Upon the Protein-to-Carbohydrate Ratio

What this graph indicates is that if you are eating more than twice as many carbohydrates as protein (a protein-to-carbohydrate ratio of less than 0.5) at a meal, you are likely to make too much insulin, which can lead to increased fat accumulation. On the other hand, if you eating more protein than carbohydrate (a protein-to-carbohydrate ratio greater than 1.0) at a meal, you are likely to make too much of the hormone glucagon, which can lead to ketosis. Don't worry about these numbers, because if you use the eye and palm method described in Chapter 3, you should always be within these limits and therefore in the Zone.

The reason I show this graph is to indicate that there is a mathematical foundation for the Zone, and that you can fine-tune each of the meals you like to eat to always be in the Zone, just as you would adjust the carburetor in your car.

You may want even greater precision (especially for adjusting your hormonal carburetor), and there are two additional food accounting methods that I have found to be useful over the years.

THE ZONE "1–2–3" METHOD

Since many Americans are already accustomed to reading the nutritional labels on food, I have developed an easy-to-use system for building Zone meals. Rather than counting calories, however, you'll be counting grams of fat, protein, and carbohydrates. For packaged food, you can take a quick look at the food label to see how many grams of each macronutrient it contains. Some foods will contain proteins, carbohydrates, and fats in various combinations, but normally most will contain a bulk amount of just one of these three. And what about foods that aren't packaged or labeled, such as fresh meats, produce, and even bagels? You can quickly learn the carbohydrate, protein, and fat content of these types of foods by turning to Appendix B at the back of this book.

How do you actually use the 1–2–3 method? It's just as it sounds: for every *one* gram of fat you consume, you want to add *two* grams of low-fat protein and *three* grams of carbohydrate to every meal. Let's go back to the typical American female who needs about 3 ounces of low-fat protein at each meal. This is about 20 grams of protein. Therefore, her typical Zone meal would consist of 10 grams of fat, 20 grams of protein, and 30 grams of carbohydrates, or "1–2–3." The typical American male, who needs 4 ounces of low-fat protein at each meal, would eat about 30 grams of protein. Therefore, his typical Zone meal would contain about 15 grams of fat, 30 grams of protein, and 45 grams of carbohydrate, or again, "1–2–3."

Just to go through the math again, take the number of grams of protein you plan to consume (like 30) and divide it by 2 to give the number of fat grams.

30 grams of protein ÷ 2 = 15 grams of fat

Then take the number of fat grams (15) and add to the number of protein grams (30) to get the number of carbohydrate grams (45) for that meal as shown below:

30 grams of protein + 15 grams of fat = 45 grams of carbohydrate

This simple accounting system gives a protein-to-carbohydrate ratio of 0.7, about midway in the Zone as shown in the previous graph. These numbers are by no means set in concrete. They can be altered to your particular biochemistry. But by following this system, you can make adjustments to the Zone Diet with a high degree of precision. So let's see how the "1–2–3" system works in practice.

Protein

Here is a helpful hint for helping to better visualize what 20 to 30 grams of protein actually represents: Get an inexpensive kitchen scale, and then measure out 3 ounces of low-fat animal protein or 4½ ounces of fish. This would provide 20 grams of protein, suitable for most females. For males, measure out 4 ounces of low-fat animal protein or 6 ounces of fish. This would represent what 30 grams of protein looks like. Within a few days, you can eye these amounts at home, in restaurants, and at dinner parties. You'll soon realize that these amounts of protein are what you generally get at the most exclusive French restaurants.

Carbohydrates

Let's take a closer look at carbohydrates. When you read a food label, it lists the grams of total carbohydrate. However, that number also includes the grams of fiber, which has no effect on insulin. So to get an indication of the effect of a particular carbohydrate source on insulin stimulation, you have to subtract the fiber content. In the following table I show you the amount of insulin-stimulating carbohydrates in several typical food items.

Amounts of Insulin-Stimulating Carbohydrates in Various Foods

Food	Volume	Total Carbs (G)	Fiber (G)	Insulin-Stimulating Carbs (G)
Pasta	1 cup	40	2	38
Apple	1 medium	20	4	16
Broccoli	1 cup	7	4	3

You can quickly see that you would have to eat a tremendous volume of broccoli (approximately 12 cups) to consume the same amount of carbohydrates as eating a relatively small amount of cooked pasta. This is why starches, breads, and grains are considered high-density carbohydrates, whereas fruits are considered medium-density carbohydrates, and vegetables are considered low-density carbohydrates. The Zone Diet relies heavily on low-density carbohydrates, so large volumes of food must be consumed in order to have an appreciable impact on insulin. On the other hand, very small volumes of high-density carbohydrate stimulate excess insulin, which is why they are used in moderation in the Zone.

There is also a lot of confusion about simple and complex carbohydrates. In reality, all carbohydrates must be broken down into simple carbohydrates to be absorbed. The rate at which any carbohydrate enters the bloodstream as the simple sugar glucose is known as the *glycemic index.*

It turns out that some complex carbohydrates such as potatoes, rice, and carrots actually enter the bloodstream as glucose at a faster rate than does table sugar! As a result, the simple distinction of simple and complex carbohydrates is not of great use in helping you control insulin.

As I describe in greater detail in my upcoming book *The Soy Zone*, the key to understanding the effect of any carbohydrate source on insulin is not related to its glycemic index, but to its glycemic load. The concept of glycemic load takes into account both the density of carbohydrates in a given food volume and also their rate of entry into the bloodstream.

So now we can redefine a favorable carbohydrate as one that has a low glycemic load. The lower the glycemic load, the more favorable the carbohydrate choice is for the Zone, as shown below.

FAVORABLE AND UNFAVORABLE CARBOHYDRATES

Favorable (have a lower effect on insulin)
Most vegetables (except corn and carrots)
Most fruits (except bananas and raisins)
Selected grains (oatmeal and barley)

Unfavorable (have a greater effect on insulin)
Grains and starches (pasta, bread, bagels, cereals, potatoes, etc.)
Selected fruits (bananas, raisins, etc.)
Selected vegetables (corn and carrots)

If you are following the "1–2–3" program, the typical female would need to eat approximately 30 grams of carbohydrate at a meal, whereas the typical male would consume about 45 grams of carbohydrates at a meal. Listed below are the food amounts that supply 10 grams of carbohydrates.

Food Volumes That Supply 10 Grams of Carbohydrates

Food	Volume
Broccoli	3 cups
String beans	1 cup
Apple	½
Strawberries	1 cup
Pasta	¼ cup
Rice	⅓ cup
Bread	½ slice

So to supply 30 grams of carbohydrate for a Zone meal for a typical female, one could choose 1 cup of strawberries (10 grams), 1 cup of string beans (10 grams), and half a piece of bread (10 grams). This would supply 30 grams of carbohydrate, enough to balance 20 grams of protein. For a Zone meal for the typical male, he might have 1½ cups of broccoli (5 grams), 1 cup of strawberries (10 grams), an apple (20 grams), and ¼ cup of pasta (10 grams). This would provide 45 grams of carbohydrate, enough to balance 30 grams of protein. Mix and match your carbohydrates any way you want as long as they don't overwhelm the protein content of the meal.

As you can see from this example, it's not that you can never eat unfavorable carbohydrates; just treat them as condiments and use them in moderation.

Fats

The primary fat you will be adding to the Zone is monounsaturated fat. But keep in mind that the Zone is not a program of fat gluttony. Following the "1–2–3" method, the typical female would need about 10 grams of fat in a Zone meal, and the typical male would require about 15 grams. Listed below are some monounsaturated fat choices that when added to the protein content of a Zone meal will provide a total of 10 grams of fat.

Again, mix and match your fats to match your protein and carbohydrate amounts as long as you don't overconsume them.

Monounsaturated Fat Choices That Provide a Total of 10 Grams of Fat in a Typical Zone Meal

Food	Volume
Olive oil	1½ teaspoons
Guacamole	4 tablespoons
Slivered almonds	2 tablespoons
Almonds	12
Macadamia nuts	2

So our Zone meal for a typical female might have 1½ teaspoons of olive oil (in a vinegar and olive oil dressing), providing a total of 10 grams of monounsaturated fat. The typical male Zone meal might have 2 tablespoons of slivered almonds (10 grams) and 2 tablespoons of guacamole (5 grams), providing a total of 15 grams of monounsaturated fat. Even though you are adding fat to the Zone, it is still a low-fat program (in terms of fat grams), and more important, one that is very low in saturated fat.

So let's now look at the typical Zone meal for a female or male.

Typical Female Zone Meal | ### Typical Male Zone Meal

Protein

Typical Female Zone Meal	Typical Male Zone Meal
3 ounces chicken breast	4 ounces chicken breast

Carbohydrates

1 cup strawberries	1½ cups broccoli
1 cup string beans	1 cup strawberries
½ piece bread	1 apple
¼ cup pasta	

Fat

1½ teaspoons olive oil	2 tablespoons slivered almonds
	2 tablespoons guacamole

Each meal follows the "1–2–3" method, and you can see that no one is going to be deprived by either meal, even though the typical female Zone meal was less than 300 calories and the typical male Zone meal was slightly over 400 calories. Eat three similar-sized meals each day plus two Zone snacks, and your caloric intake is approximately 1,200 for a female and about 1,500 for a male. The Zone Diet is a lifetime program of reduced calories, but without deprivation (because of the large size of the meals) or hunger (because blood sugar levels are being maintained at a constant level).

ZONE FOOD BLOCKS

The other food accounting system that I developed is called Zone Food Blocks. Many people find this system easier to use than the "1–2–3" method, but it does take a little getting used to. Basically, it measures food in blocks rather than in grams.

Personally, I believe that Zone Food Blocks are ultimately easier because you don't have to remember as many numbers as with the "1–2–3" method. Zone Food Blocks are volumes or weights of various food sources that contain the same number of grams in pre-measured blocks of protein, carbohydrate, and fat. Now all you have to do is maintain those Zone Food Blocks in a 1:1:1 ratio to be squarely in the center of the Zone.

With the Zone Food Block method, one block of protein is equal to 7 grams, one block of carbohydrate is equal to 9 grams, and one block of fat is equal to 3 grams. This means that the typical American female will require 3 Zone Food Blocks each of protein, carbohydrate, and fat at each meal, whereas the typical American male would require 4 Zone Food Blocks of each at every meal.

Since people generally only eat 20 different food items, all you have to do is remember what the Zone Food Block sizes are for your favorite foods. Actually, remembering your telephone number is probably more difficult. Appendix C lists many of the most common foods, broken down into Zone Food Blocks. This is also the system described in my other books, including *The Zone* and *Zone-Perfect Meals in Minutes*.

ADJUSTING YOUR HORMONAL CARBURETOR

Is there one diet for everyone? The answer is both yes and no. There is one hormonally correct diet for everyone, and that is one that keeps insulin within the Zone. However, the balance of protein to carbohydrate to reach the Zone might be different from person to person, and we obviously don't all like to eat the same things. Whether you are using the eye and palm method, the "1–2–3" method, or the Zone Food Block method, the technique for adjusting your hormonal carburetor is essentially the same.

So how do you know if your last meal was hormonally correct? It's very simple. After you eat, look at your watch. Then, four hours later, ask yourself two questions:

Are you hungry?

Do you have good mental focus?

If the answer to both these questions is yes, then you know your last meal was hormonally correct, based on your biochemistry. You can always go back to that same exact meal in the exact same proportions to get the exact same hormonal output. Just like a drug. All you need is to create 10 hormonally winning meals (2 breakfasts, 3 lunches, and 5 dinners) that you can constantly rotate in your diet.

On the other hand, if the answer to either question is no, then you know your last meal was not hormonally correct. For example, if you are hungry and loopy (like after eating a big bowl of pasta), this means that you consumed too much carbohydrate relative to protein in your last meal, and pushed your insulin too high. Plan to have the same meal again, and keep the protein constant but reduce the carbohydrates by about 10 grams or one Zone Block of carbohydrate.

If you have a good mental focus but you are hungry, that's an indication that you had too much protein relative to carbohydrate. As a result, you pushed your insulin too low, so the brain is telling you to eat again, even though the brain is getting adequate blood sugar. If this is the case, next time you have that same meal, keep the protein constant, but increase the amount of carbohydrate by about 10 grams or one Zone Block of carbohydrate. By using either food accounting system, you are learning how to adjust your hormonal carburetor to your own unique biochemistry and using only the foods you like to eat.

CAN YOU EVER BE TOO THIN?

The Zone is designed to bring you to your ideal body weight and keep you there for a lifetime. However, you can become too lean. How do you know if you've reached this point? You'll be able to see your abdominal muscles. Usually this is only a problem for elite athletes, and may occur when one includes intensive exercise to the Zone. But if it does happen (God forbid, who would want to look like an Olympic athlete?), then what do you do? You don't want to add any protein to your diet because it is already protein-adequate. You don't want to add any more carbohydrate to your diet, since that would raise insulin levels. So there's only one nutrient left to add to your diet that has calories, but has no effect on insulin. It's our old friend fat, and in particular monounsaturated fat. Add more monounsaturated fat to your diet (such as olive oil, macadamia nuts, or guacamole) to give you enough calories to maintain your percentage of body fat at a level consistent with good health. Actually, many of the elite athletes I work with consume more than 50 percent of the calories as monounsaturated fat to maintain their percentage of body fat in the appropriate range for optimal sports performance. Should your body fat begin to increase too much, then cut back on the amount of extra monounsaturated fat added to your diet until your abdominal muscles begin to reappear.

THE ONCE-A-MONTH PORKY PIG MEAL

The Zone Diet is not restrictive, nor does it require perfect attention. In fact, you will get 75 percent of the benefits of the Zone by following it 75 percent of the time. As a result, there is no guilt on the Zone. If you have a bad meal, just make sure that your next meal is squarely in the Zone. No one is perfect, nor should anyone ever become obsessive regarding the preparation of Zone meals.

And even if you were perfect, I strongly recommend eating a

large carbohydrate meal (pasta, Mexican food, and so on) at least once a month, just so you can feel miserable the next day. You will be bloated, fatigued, mentally foggy—basically the feeling of being hit by a Mack truck. What you are suffering from is an insulin hangover. The reason why I recommend such torture once a month is to reinforce how powerful food can be, and that only one hormonally incorrect meal can send you directly to carbohydrate hell. It's okay, because your next meal will take you back to the Zone. Unfortunately, some of us need some powerful reinforcement from time to time to reaffirm how we want to spend the rest of our lives.

If you want to be even more precise (because, after all, the Zone is based on science), then I recommend that you read my books *Mastering the Zone* and *Zone-Perfect Meals in Minutes* for more detailed information on how to adjust your current diet to make it more hormonally correct.

12

SUCCESS STORIES FROM THE ZONE

Being in the Zone will help you think better, perform better, and look better. But the power of this dietary technology goes far beyond these benefits alone. It was developed to treat what I call "either/or" medical conditions, medical conditions that either have no treatment or those for which the treatments are less than desirable.

Hormonal control will be the key to twenty-first-century medicine, and much of this hormonal control comes from the food that you eat. You can take advantage of this fact when you enter the Zone. The end result is that some very remarkable changes are possible if you treat food with the same respect that you treat a prescription drug.

While I can tell you this over and over, perhaps you would like to hear what other people have to say about the Zone and how it has affected their lives. These are their stories. They may begin like yours, or like the story of someone you know. Their endings, however, come straight from the Zone.

Consider the story of Willard H., a prostate cancer survivor who wrote:

I just returned from the Mayo Clinic, where I go for my annual physical. All of my tests came out well. My PSA [a marker for prostate cancer] is undetectable. My cholesterol has continued to decrease from 210 to 150. Thanks and congratulations go to you and the Zone. I spoke with my physicians about the Zone. They were not experts on nutrition, but said they thought it was a good program.

Neither their encouragement nor discouragement would have made a difference with me. I'm on your program for life. I give a lot of credit to your program for keeping my PSA at the bottom end of the scale.

Now, five years later, Willard H. continues to write to me about his continuing good health and virtually zero PSA levels.

Reaching the Zone is all about improved quality of life. That's why I particularly like the letter that I got from Joan S., a multiple sclerosis patient, who wrote:

This "incurable" multiple sclerosis is reversing after sixteen years. It feels like I'm living a miracle. I'm glad I've kept daily notes, because it seems unbelievable. I keep pinching myself.

What is even more encouraging are letters from individuals who have been on medication for decades, like Audrey, who wrote me the following:

I have suffered from clinical depression for 37 years and spent thousands of dollars on therapy and medication. Plagued by weight gain and other side effects from the antidepressants, I became deter- mined to go off the medications altogether. Working with my doctor, I have been medication free for 4 months, and my depression still has not returned. Before I heard about the Zone, I cut out sugar and alcohol. Last month, I heard about the Zone from a friend and decided to try it. I've found that I'm happier and able to think more clearly than I can ever remember. (I never thought that it was possi- ble to feel this way.) What's more, the Zone has been able to reverse the lingering effects of the antidepressants. Before I went on the Zone, I was 140 pounds–25 pounds above what I used to weigh. Now I can happily report that I weigh 125 and can get into my favorite clothes! The Zone is helping me in so many areas of my life, especially phys- ically and psychologically. When these two areas are stable, the rest of life just flows.

Another condition that responds rapidly to the Zone is high blood pressure, as Steve W. wrote:

I tried your program and am very satisfied. My blood pressure was 132/103. Even after cutting out desserts and having my weight drop to 172, my blood pressure had not changed. After 45 days on the Zone, my weight is in the low 160s and my blood pressure has dropped to 103/73. I guess you can say you probably saved my life. I am sorry I had to give up so many of my favorite things, such as bread, pizza, and rice. But I am developing new favorites, such as cherries, peaches, blueberries, turkey breast and more. I guess it's a small price to pay to live longer.

I also received a letter from Pat G., who wrote:

I weighed 205 pounds and was a Type 2 diabetic. My brain was always foggy from the use of my medications. After 4 months on the Zone, I have lost 41 pounds, and I feel great. My body is still changing. My muscles are building and becoming more toned while I am losing fat. I take no medications. My blood sugar levels continue to remain in the normal range. I have very little if any pain now from my back and my leg. My doctor can't believe it.

Pat's experience in the Zone and improved control of blood sugar is no different from that of lots of other people including Fedore L., who wrote,

During the month of September, I developed a strange taste of sawdust in my mouth and some needle-like pain in my liver, in addition to a small amount of foam in my urine. I decided to go to my doctor, and my blood tests of October 13 showed a fasting blood glucose level of 288, and inflammation of the liver. He prescribed a medication for diabetes, then asked me to come back in 6 weeks for another test. I seriously pondered whether to try the Zone and not the medication. I reported it to my doctor who, as expected, was not at all pleased. I bargained with him for four weeks of a trial. I confessed to him that I had abused my body for the last 40 years (I'm now 71), therefore wanted to give my body a chance for recovery. Scared to death, I followed the Zone to the letter. Four weeks later, my blood glucose test was 103, totally normal. Then, on purpose, I exited the

Zone a bit, and a week later my blood sugar had risen to 126. I am truly feeling that food must be perceived as a drug.

Relief from pain is crucial for one's quality of life. That's why I was happy to receive a letter from Belinda D. Belinda is a health care professional who was not only overweight, but also suffered from repetitive stress injuries that had required three separate surgeries. She was still taking 18 aspirin per day to ease the pain. Belinda wrote:

When I picked up your book in the bookstore, my first response was to put it back on the shelf and renew my promise not to try a diet program. What made me stop and buy the book was the section I read on chronic pain and arthritis. At that point, I was ready to try anything. Within a month of following the Zone, my pain levels were reduced to a point where I stopped taking all medication, and I was actually returning to basically pain-free living. The weight loss I have experienced has been an added bonus to the way I feel. For the record I have lost 40 pounds in the last five months. I have a way to go, but I feel no stress in getting to my ideal weight. My husband has been equally as successful in the Zone. He has returned to his ideal weight of 178 (from 220), and it is like having a new man around the house. The biggest improvement has come in his emotional well being. Thank you again for your work and for publishing the information in such a clear and concise manner.

There are many more stories like these, but I feel that the examples I have chosen are representative of my basic concept that food is a very powerful drug if used correctly.

But what about overweight individuals who exercise to lose weight? Consider Steve G., who three years ago weighed 313 pounds. Determined to change his life, Steve started biking and running 1½ hours per day and sticking to a 1,000-calorie diet rich in carbohydrates and low in fat. Within a year, he had reached 250. For the next year and a half, he did the same exercise and low-calorie, high-carbohydrate diet and nothing happened. His weight remained the same. As he wrote:

I noticed your book this past summer one day in a bookstore, and could not believe what perfect sense you made. I actually cut back on some of my exercise and added more fat to my diet. I applied your technology and the weight has been dropping off. I'm down to 205 now, and headed toward my ultimate goal of 174. On top of it all, I feel energized, whereas on every other diet, I always felt very drained. The Zone simply works.

Obviously, I am very gratified when I receive such letters, testimonials, and profound thanks from people whose lives have been dramatically improved by the Zone program. The real credit does not go to me, however, but to these readers. They took the initiative to change their own lives, and you can, too. I hope that some of these stories illustrate the potential of the Zone Diet to transform your health, and perhaps will inspire some changes of your own. Remember, the Zone Diet is not radical; it just requires you to look at food in a new way and take responsibility when you eat—a small price to pay for a longer and better life.

13

FREQUENTLY ASKED QUESTIONS

GENERAL

Why are both protein and carbohydrates required at every meal and snack?

Zone logic says that excess insulin will make you fat and keep you fat. Your goal is to maintain insulin in a Zone, not too high, not too low, throughout the day. The protein and carbohydrate content of a meal has a dramatic impact on insulin production and determines how well you keep insulin in that Zone for the next four to six hours.

Why is meal timing so important?

As with a medication, you want to control the body's utilization of protein and carbohydrate consistently throughout the day, and you should eat a minimum of three meals and two snacks. A Zone meal should provide you with four to six hours in the Zone, whereas a snack is good for approximately two to two and a half hours. Additionally, you must eat within one hour after waking, and don't forget your afternoon and late-night snacks. Eating every five hours, whether you're hungry or not, is necessary to stay in the Zone. In fact, lack of hunger without cravings for sugars and sweets coupled with good mental focus is a good indicator that you're in the Zone.

Like planning your daily activities, meal and snack times should be planned accordingly. Based on your wake-up time, determine those timepoints throughout the day when it's time to eat your next meal or snack.

If I follow the Zone Diet, does this mean I can never have rice, pasta, or bagels again?

No, but you should be using these carbohydrate sources in moderation, like condiments. Simply make sure that most of your daily intake of carbohydrates comes from vegetables and fruits and, whenever possible, cut down on your intake of grains and starches.

I thought complex carbohydrates (such as grains and starches) were good for you.

Grains and starches are high-density carbohydrates that are very easy to overconsume, which will elevate insulin. As an example, one cup of cooked pasta has the same amount of carbohydrates as 12 cups of broccoli. Low-density carbohydrates in the form of fruits and vegetables are virtually impossible to overeat, and their fiber content slows the entry rates of carbohydrates into the bloodstream and helps control insulin levels. In addition, don't forget that fruits and vegetables are loaded with vitamins and minerals, unlike grains and starches. Remember, it's not that you'll never consume grains and starches again, but when you do, they must be consumed in moderation, compared to fruits and vegetables.

Do I have to be obsessive about the Zone Diet to be successful?

No. Obviously, the greater the precision, the greater the results, but even if you only play by the general rules of the Zone and use the eye and palm method, you won't be too far away from the center of the Zone. Just remember to pay very close attention to your hunger and mental focus four to six hours after a meal. Using your eyes, you will be able to adjust your hormonal carburetor with increasing precision without having to obsess about portion size, grams, or calculations.

Isn't the Zone Diet a high-protein diet?

No, it's a protein-adequate diet. You should never eat excessive amounts of protein, nor should you consume any less than your body requires. At each meal, an adequate amount of protein is approximately 3 ounces for the typical female and 4 ounces for the typical male. Both snacks should contain one ounce of protein. These amounts of low-fat protein are hardly considered excessive.

I prefer to eat smaller, more frequent meals throughout the day. Is it possible to stay in the Zone?

Actually, the greater the number of small meals you eat, the better the insulin control. This is called *grazing*.

Should I be concerned about such a seemingly low daily caloric intake?

For most females the minimum total calories consumed is 1,100 to 1,200 calories per day, and for most males, the calories consumed is 1,400 to 1,500. While this might seem like a deprivation diet that leaves you constantly fatigued, the Zone Diet will actually eliminate hunger between meals, without the nagging cravings for sugars and sweets, while maintaining peak physical and mental energy throughout the day.

You aren't hungry, because the balance of protein to carbohydrate maintains stable blood sugar levels to the brain. Finally, on the Zone Diet, you are eating as if you are already at your ideal body weight because you are using a combination of your stored body fat and incoming calories to meet your daily caloric requirements. Therefore, once you achieve your ideal weight, you don't change your diet at all.

Doesn't any low-calorie diet cause fat loss? (A calorie is a calorie.)

Not necessarily. Research studies in the 1950s demonstrated this with several different diets consisting of 1,000 calories per day. All patients lost substantial weight on a high-protein (90% of calories) diet, high-fat (90% of calories) diet, and mixed (42% of calories as carbohydrate) diet, but most patients actually gained weight on a high-carbohydrate (90% of calories) diet. Cutting back on calories without lowering your insulin levels is a surefire prescription for feelings of deprivation, constant hunger, fatigue, and, finally, failure. Any time you reduce calories, you will lose some weight, but eventually you hit a hormonal plateau where the weight loss (and, more important, fat loss) stops, but feelings of hunger, deprivation, and fatigue continue. Unlike other reduced-calorie dietary programs, the Zone Diet is a hormonal control program that maintains adequate levels of blood sugar to the brain, which allows for significant calorie reduction without hunger, fatigue, or deprivation. This lifelong use of the Zone makes it the only "drug" that can successfully provide permanent fat loss.

How long will it be before I can expect to see results on the Zone Diet?

Within two to three days you should see a noticeable reduction in your carbohydrate cravings and an increased mental focus. Within five days you will notice a significant decrease in hunger throughout the day coupled with greater physical performance and less fatigue as the day wears on. Keep in mind that this is a fat loss program; don't expect rapid weight loss, which is often mostly water. The maximum fat loss you can expect, no matter how strictly you follow the program or how much you exercise, is one to one and a half pounds of fat per week. It is simply impossible to reduce excess body fat any faster on any dietary program. Within two weeks, you will notice that your clothes are fitting much better. Judge your success by the fit of your clothes and not by changes on your bathroom scale.

What is the minimum amount of daily protein intake?

I always recommend a minimum of 75 grams of protein throughout the day for adults. This is ideal for most women, whereas most men will require about 100 grams of low-fat protein each day.

Won't the Zone Diet cause osteoporosis and kidney failure?

The Zone is a protein-adequate diet in which small amounts of protein are portioned evenly throughout the day. No one should eat more protein than their body requires, but conversely, no one should eat less, because you will put yourself in a state of protein malnutrition. On the Zone Diet, you are not only eating adequate protein, but also spreading it over three meals and two snacks. It's almost as if you are receiving an intravenous drip of protein throughout the day. The newest research actually indicates that women who eat more protein have 70 percent fewer hip fractures than those who eat less than 75 grams per day. Furthermore, the additional research indicates that even for patients with kidney failure, earlier reports about protein restriction may have been overblown. And if you don't have kidney failure there is no evidence that eating the amounts of recommended protein in the Zone Diet has any negative effects.

Why don't the French have high rates of heart disease?

Nutritionists just hate the French. They smoke, they drink, they eat lots of fat, they don't exercise, they seem to have a very good time, and they have the lowest rates of heart disease in Europe. It's called the French Paradox. It's only a paradox if the results are contrary to your expectations. Obviously, there are a number of reasons for these surprising statistics, but I believe the major factor is that their meals are moderate in calories, rich in fruits and vegetables, always contain protein, and include fat. That's also a good definition of the Zone. Then there is the so-called Spanish Paradox. In the last 20 years, Spaniards have eaten more protein, more fat, and fewer grains, and their rates of cardiovascular disease are dropping.

The Chinese eat a lot of rice; don't they have low rates of heart disease?

No. According to the American Heart Association the rates of cardiovascular disease in urban Chinese males are nearly as great as in American males, and Chinese females, both rural and urban, actually have greater rates of cardiovascular disease than American females. In addition, the data from the American Heart Association indicate that the Chinese have greater overall adult mortality than is found in Americans. These data demonstrate the danger of using epidemiological data to make far-reaching dietary assumptions.

I'm concerned about pesticides on fruits and vegetables, and the hormones and antibiotics used in beef and chicken production. What should I do?

These are valid concerns. You should always try to eat organic fruits, vegetables, and range-fed beef and chicken. However, be prepared to pay a significantly higher price and to cope with their scarcity. Don't, however, make this an excuse for not eating the appropriate protein-to-carbohydrate balance at every meal.

I'm not overweight. Why would I need to follow the Zone Diet?

The Zone is not a diet. It's a lifelong hormonal control program. Loss of excess body fat is only a pleasant and very desirable side benefit. The important reason to follow the Zone Diet is that it is the only dietary program which has been demonstrated to reverse the aging process. Although the Zone Diet was originally developed for cardiovascular patients, it was extensively tested on world-class athletes. Between those two extremes lies everyone else. If you are at your ideal weight and want to think better, perform better, and live longer, then the Zone Diet is for you.

Can I continue taking my vitamins and minerals?

Vitamins and minerals are an excellent low-cost insurance policy to ensure adequate micronutrient (vitamins and minerals) intake. However, the Zone Diet—which is primarily composed of low-fat protein, fruits, and vegetables—provides an excellent source of vitamins and minerals, and requires much less supplementation. The only supplements that I strongly recommend are fish oils and extra Vitamin E.

What exactly do you mean by "use in moderation" when referring to unfavorable carbohydrates?

Try not to make unfavorable carbohydrates (grains, starches, breads, and pasta) more than 25 percent of the total carbohydrate grams in a meal. Use them as condiments, not as your primary carbohydrate source.

Should I be concerned about sodium?

Not if you are following the Zone Diet, because excess insulin activates another hormonal system that promotes sodium retention. However, it always makes sense not to use excessive amounts of sodium.

I'm a pure vegetarian. How can I make this diet work for me?

Simply add protein-rich vegetarian foods to your current diet to maintain the correct protein-to-carbohydrate ratio. Ideal choices would be firm and extra-firm tofu and isolated soybean protein powder. The new generation of soybean-based meat substitutes (hot dogs, hamburgers, sausages, and so on) is another excellent way of turning a carbohydrate-rich vegetarian diet into a vegetarian Zone diet. Traditional vegetarian protein sources, such as beans, have an exceptionally high amount of carbohydrate for the amount of protein they provide, which makes it impossible to achieve the desired protein-to-carbohydrate balance to enter the Zone.

Which protein powders are best?

Sources of isolated protein include egg and milk combinations and lactose-free whey powder. For vegetarians, isolated soy protein powders are excellent choices. Protein powders are available at most health food stores. Protein powders can be added to any carbohydrate-rich meal, like oatmeal, to make them more hormonally favorable. They can also be added to flours and mixes (like pancake, muffin, and cookie mixes) for cooking and baking to fortify the protein content.

What impact will various cooking methods have on the quality of macronutrients or micronutrients?

Cooking has little effect on macronutrients (except that excessive heat can damage and cross-link protein with carbohydrates). However, cooking can have a very negative effect on micronutrients (vitamins and minerals). Vitamins are extraordinarily sensitive to heat. In addition, minerals can be leached out of food when cooked with water. Therefore, steaming vegetables is an ideal way to retain micronutrients, yet make the vegetables more digestible. Fruits are usually eaten raw, retaining all of their micronutrients. The more carbohydrates are processed or cooked, the more rapid their entry rate into the bloodstream. This is why "instant" forms of carbohydrate like one-minute rice or instant potatoes should be avoided.

Should I eat my Zone meal or snack even if I'm not hungry?

Yes. This is the best time to eat in order to maintain insulin equilibrium from one meal to the next. If you're thinking hormonally, you want to maintain insulin in a Zone by eating every five hours. As with an IV drip, you want to control the entry rates of protein and carbohydrate evenly throughout the day. That's why everyone should consume three meals and two snacks each day.

Will this diet heal the damage done to my body over the years?

The body has a remarkable ability to repair itself, given the appropriate tools. The best of those tools is the diet, especially one that orchestrates the desired hormonal responses that accelerate the repair process.

Why don't I count all the protein, carbohydrate, and fat in everything I eat?

Because you would need a mini-computer to make all the calculations. This is why I recommend the eye and palm method to balance your plate. If you want more precision, then you can use either the "1–2–3" or Zone Food Block methods.

Will a liquid meal in the correct ratio get me to the Zone?

A liquid meal has a much greater surface area than solid food. Therefore, the digestion and entry rate of macronutrients into the bloodstream cannot be controlled that well, and there is a corresponding decrease in the desired hormonal control. Liquid meals are more convenient but hormonally not as desirable as solid food.

They can be used occasionally if you just don't have the time to cook, and are much more desirable than skipping a meal or snack.

Can children use the Zone?

The diet is ideal for children because they need to be in the Zone even more than adults do. The average preadolescent child (boy or girl) will need about 15 grams of protein per meal, with the appropriate amounts of fat and carbohydrate. After puberty, children should eat the same amounts as a typical adult. The one protein source that virtually every child will eat is string cheese. Although a little high in saturated fat, string cheese is a good way to introduce more protein into your child's diet. That leaves just the hard part for parents: getting your kids to eat fruits and vegetables instead of pasta and bread.

How do I know that two years from now the Zone Diet will not turn out to be like the other diets that initially produce great results?

First, the Zone is not a diet, but a lifelong hormonal control program that allows you to maximize your full genetic potential. Second, the Zone has been in the popular press for more than five years, and the newest research has confirmed everything I originally stated when *The Zone* was first published in 1995. Most important, the hormonal systems the Zone Diet is based upon have evolved over the last 40 million years and are unlikely to change soon. Many fad diets are based on gluttony and extremism. Either they let you eat all the carbohydrates you want (high-carbohydrate, low-fat diets) or all the protein and fat you want (high-protein diets), and neither type worries about the quantities consumed. The Zone Diet is based on balance (of protein and carbohydrate) and moderation (of calories), with limits on the amount of protein, carbohydrate, and fat consumed at every meal.

What if I make a mistake or go overboard?

Don't worry, you're only temporarily knocked out of the Zone. You can get back on track with your next meal or snack. Zone living is guilt-free.

I'm currently taking medications. How will this affect the Zone Diet?

Any change in diet (for better or worse) will affect the metabolism of the drug(s) you are taking. Always consult with a physician before starting the Zone Diet or any other dietary plan. In addition, many medications will actually raise insulin levels, making it difficult to enjoy the desired benefits no matter how strictly you follow the program. See if your physician could possibly switch you to a medication that does not negatively influence insulin levels. However, never change the dosage or stop taking your medication without first consulting your physician.

I haven't exercised in years. Should I?

Since you are not fatigued or listless on the Zone Diet, you may be inclined to start an exercise program for the first time in years. While not as important as your diet, exercise does play an important role in helping you control insulin levels. The best form of exercise is any routine you will perform on a regular basis. If you haven't exercised for a long time, building up to a brisk 30-minute walk is a great way to get started again. As your endurance builds, you may wish to increase the intensity and even add some form of weight training as part of your regular workout schedule. Never think that increased exercise can erase the problems associated with poor diet. I use the 80/20 rule: 80 percent of your ability to control insulin will come from the diet and 20 percent from exercise.

I exercise on a regular basis at high intensity. How can I optimize my workout schedule to get the maximum hormonal bang for the buck?

Whether you are training with weights or training aerobically, eat a Zone snack 30 minutes prior to exercise. This will set the hormonal stage to trigger the preferential burning of stored body fat as soon as your workout begins. Have another Zone snack within 30 minutes after the training session ends and a Zone meal no more than 2 hours later. Most important of all, don't forget your bedtime snack.

I get confused when it comes to the difference between proteins and carbohydrates. Are there any simple rules to help me when I shop?

Here is a simple rule for distinguishing between protein and carbohydrates: Protein moves around (or at least once did) and carbohydrates come from the ground, in the form of grains (pasta, breads, and cereals), vegetables, and fruits. When shopping, always try to stick to the periphery of the market. There you will find fresh fruits and vegetables, the deli case, the salad bar, and the meat department. Down the middle aisles, you'll find all the packaged carbohydrates, a surefire way to increase insulin levels and knock you out of the Zone.

What about alcohol?

The body treats alcohol as if it were a carbohydrate. For all intents and purposes, treat 4 ounces of wine, a bottle of beer, or 1½ ounces of distilled liquor as if it were 10 grams of carbohydrate or one Zone block of carbohydrate.

As long as my protein and carbohydrate balance at any meal or snack is based on Zone guidelines, couldn't I eat all I wanted and still keep insulin under control?

Any excess calories that can't be used immediately by the body will be stored as fat, even if the meal is perfectly balanced, and the extra calories will also increase overall insulin levels. The typical female should consume approximately 300 calories in a meal, and the typical male should consume approximately 400.

FAT FACTS

Why do I need extra fat? What does it do?

Paradoxically, it takes fat to burn fat, especially if the fat source is monounsaturated fat. Remember, the Zone Diet is not an excuse for fat gluttony, but there is a need to add back reasonable amounts of fat to each meal. First, monounsaturated fat doesn't affect insulin and thus acts as a control rod to slow carbohydrate entry into the bloodstream, thereby reducing the insulin response. Second, it releases a hormone (cholecystokinin, or CCK) from the stomach that tells the brain to stop eating. Third, it makes food taste better. Most of your fat intake should be in the form of monounsaturated fat, and the amount of fat you consume is dictated by the amount of protein you consume at each meal. If anything, be more liberal than restrictive with your monounsaturated fat intake.

Can I lose too much body fat?

Obviously, it's possible to lose too much body fat. Once you achieve a weight and look that you are happy with, and wish to stabilize your body weight, simply add more monounsaturated fat to your Zone Diet. Since you were always eating as if you were at your ideal weight, the protein and carbohydrate content of your diet remains the same. Therefore, to prevent any further weight loss, you must add more fat, preferably monounsaturated fat, as caloric ballast to prevent any further fat loss. This extra monounsaturated fat provides the extra calories to maintain your ideal body weight without affecting insulin levels. Many world-class athletes on the Zone Diet consume more than 50 percent of their daily calories in the form of fat.

What are the best sources for long-chain omega-3 fats?

The best sources are cold-water fatty fish, such as salmon, mackerel, and sardines. Other marine sources that have a lower omega-3 fat content are common fish such as tuna, swordfish, scallops, shrimp, and lobster. Try to consume about 10 grams of long-chain omega-3 fats per week. This would translate into two servings of salmon or four servings of tuna or similar fish per week. One teaspoon of refined fish oil contains about 1 gram of long-chain omega-3 fats. Remember that your grandmother used to give you a tablespoon of cod liver oil per day? That provided about 3 grams of long-chain omega-3 fats per day, or 20 grams per week.

I'm a vegetarian and can't use fish oil. What should I do?

There is a new generation of algae-based oils that are rich in long-chain omega-3 fats. This allows the vegetarian to get adequate levels of these critical fats.

FINE-TUNING

How do I adjust my hormonal carburetor?

Not everyone is genetically the same. Your hormonal carburetor is based on the protein-to-carbohydrate balance that generates the best hormonal response for you. That hormonal response is easily measured by asking yourself, "How do I feel?" four to six hours after a meal. If you maintain excellent mental clarity and have no hunger, then the protein-to-carbohydrate balance in your last meal was ideal for your biochemistry. Your goal is to make every meal with that same ratio in order to generate the same hormonal response. For the vast majority of people, this balance is 2 grams of low-fat protein for every 3 grams of carbohydrate. So the most efficient way to fine-tune your own carburetor is to start with this ratio and then experiment slightly on either side to determine your limits by using lack of hunger and mental clarity as the parameters you wish to optimize.

I thought fat was the enemy.

Fat has no direct effect on insulin. However, monounsaturated fats like olive oil play a critical role in controlling insulin by slowing the entry rate of carbohydrates into your bloodstream. How well you control the entry rate of carbohydrates into the body determines how well you control insulin, and consequently how your body performs for the next four to six hours.

I have developed some constipation. What should I do?

A Zone Diet will switch your body to a fat-burning metabolism instead of a carbohydrate-burning metabolism. The metabolism of fat requires greater amounts of water on a daily basis. Therefore, the first step is to increase your water intake by 50 percent. If this isn't sufficient to reduce the constipation, then you are probably releasing a particular type of stored fat known as *arachidonic acid* from your fat cells. For about 25 percent of the population, there will be a transitory release of arachidonic acid. The build-up of extra arachidonic acid is a result of your previous dietary patterns. This temporary increase in arachidonic acid in the bloodstream can give rise to constipation by reducing water flow into the colon. Adding extra long-chain omega-3 fats to your diet will minimize this transitory effect. The best source of long-chain omega-3 fats is fish, but another good source is fish oil capsules, as long as the fish oil has been extensively purified. For the first week on the Zone, I recommend taking an additional 6 grams of purified fish oil per day.

How should I alter this diet if I'm pregnant or nursing my child?

If you are pregnant or nursing, you should be using the Zone to ensure adequate protein intake. For pregnant women, increase your protein intake by 10 grams at every meal, with a corresponding increase of carbohydrate and fat. In essence, you are now consuming the meals that a typical male would eat. For nursing mothers, add an extra five grams of protein and the corresponding amount of carbohydrate and fat to each Zone meal.

Can I cut back on fat intake as long as I balance my protein and carbohydrate requirements?

You can, but ironically, you will not lose as much fat. The small amount of added fat acts as a control rod to reduce the entry rate of carbohydrates into the bloodstream, thereby reducing insulin secretion. By reducing insulin, you can access your stored body fat more effectively. Also, the fat causes the release of the hormone cholecystokinin (CCK), which promotes satiety between meals. Of course, any added fat to your diet should be primarily monounsaturated fat, such as olive oil, guacamole, almonds, or macadamia nuts.

I haven't lost any weight. What am I doing wrong?

Often your weight on the scale will not change even though you are losing body fat. This is because you are likely to be gaining new lean body mass. The result is that your weight is constant, but your body composition is changing. You can tell this from the better fit of your clothes.

14

WHY HIGH-PROTEIN DIETS FAIL

High-protein diets are once again sweeping the nation: rashers of bacon and sausage in the morning, cheeseburgers (without buns) for lunch, and big steaks for dinner. Eat as much protein as you want, just don't eat any carbohydrates. And as for saturated fat, eat all you want. Sound too good to be true? Well, it is. As we grow fatter as a nation, more and more Americans are turning in desperation to these highly unbalanced diets to lose weight quickly. Unfortunately, that hope of permanent fat loss will never be realized.

First, let me make it very clear again that the Zone is *not* a high-protein diet. Although it is commonly described that way by the popular press, you now know that the Zone doesn't come close to being a high-protein diet. A high-protein diet is exactly that: you're eating excessive amounts of protein, often rich in saturated fat, at every sitting. On the Zone Diet you are *never* eating more than 3 to 4 ounces of low-fat protein at any one meal. That is exactly what every nutritionist in America recommends.

Furthermore, on the Zone Diet, you are always eating more carbohydrates than protein. In fact, while the U.S. government recommends eating three to five servings of fruits and vegetables per day, the Zone Diet recommends eating ten to fifteen servings of fruits and vegetables daily. So if the Zone Diet is not a high-protein diet, then what exactly is a high-protein diet? And more important, why have high-protein diets failed to deliver the promise of safe and permanent weight loss?

High-protein diets have been around for more than 30 years. Millions of people have tried them and lost weight. The same millions have all gained the weight back, and usually more to boot. I am one of the harshest critics of high-protein diets because I think they are unhealthy and downright dangerous. Let me explain why.

These diets tell you to eat virtually unlimited amounts of protein and fat with virtually no carbohydrates. In the absence of a minimal amount of incoming carbohydrates, the body is quickly set into an abnormal metabolic condition known as *ketosis*. This condition occurs when there is not enough carbohydrate to metabolize fat completely, and waste products known as ketone bodies begin to accumulate in the blood. In addition, without an adequate amount of incoming carbohydrates, your brain can't function properly. For this reason alone, many people on high-protein diets often feel cranky and irritable—a sure sign that their brain is malnourished for carbohydrates.

In terms of weight loss, these high-protein diets look good at first glance. Almost everyone who tries them loses weight initially. But weight loss is different from fat loss. Weight loss is a combination of loss of water, muscle, and fat. Your goal is to make sure that virtually all your weight loss comes from excess body fat. The reason behind the quick weight loss seen with high-protein diets is that your body is working overtime to expel all the ketone bodies in your system. It does this by increased urination, which in turn causes water loss. This water loss will translate into weight loss, but at the same time will leach valuable electrolytes, like potassium, from the bloodstream. This can create a false sense of accomplishment and, more seriously, lead to potentially dangerous cardiac problems. Furthermore, it has been clinically proven that both weight loss and fat loss are no different after six weeks following a high-protein diet or the Zone. So why risk potential short-term cardiac problems if the fat loss is no different from that in the Zone?

After any extended period of time, high-protein diets don't have a great track record. As you continue to diet and force your body into ketosis, insidious changes are slowly taking place in your body. First, your fat cells begin adapting themselves and become "fat magnets" that now are 10 times more active in shuttling fat into fat cells than they were before you went on the high-protein diet. This means that when you go off the diet, you'll accumulate body fat at a frightening rate. Second, your brain didn't just fall off the turnip truck. It needs blood sugar for optimal performance, which it is no longer receiving from carbohydrates. Desperate, it instructs your body to start tearing down protein in existing muscle mass to convert into glucose for energy. This is why people who stay on high-protein diets for a long period of time have that very gaunt look in the face and start losing their hair. The body is actually stripping protein from these sites to make adequate glucose levels for the brain. Third, you are consuming far too much saturated fat. This not only makes you more prone to heart disease, but makes your cells less responsive to insulin. This in turn forces the body to start making more insulin, which is what made you fat in the first place. Finally, new evidence indicates that continued ketosis leads to increased oxidation of your lipids, an important factor in the development of heart disease. These are the biochemical reasons why high-protein diets ultimately fail, and why the millions who have lost weight on them have gained their weight back and more while risking their cardiovascular health. It has happened for the last 30 years, and it will continue to happen for the next 30 years and beyond.

To further illustrate the differences between the Zone Diet and a typical high-protein diet, we can look at what a typical day might consist of for the average American male.

COMPARISON OF A HIGH-PROTEIN DIET TO THE ZONE

High-Protein	Zone
	Breakfast
Eggs, scrambled or fried	8-egg white omelet with
Bacon	2 teaspoons olive oil
Ham	1 cup slow-cooked oatmeal
Sausage	1 cup strawberries
	Lunch
Bacon cheeseburger without bun	Chicken Caesar salad with 4 oz chicken and 1 tablespoon olive-oil-and-vinegar dressing
Small tossed salad	2 cups steamed vegetables
	1 apple

Afternoon snack

None   1 oz turkey breast
                                        1 kiwi
                                        3 almonds

Dinner

Shrimp cocktail   6 oz grilled salmon covered
                                          with 2 tablespoons slivered
                                          almonds
Clear consommé   4 cups steamed vegetables
Tossed salad   1 cup mixed berries
Diet Jell-O

Late night snack

None   4 oz red wine
                                        1 oz low-fat cheese

If you take the daily consumption of protein, carbohydrate, and fat for each of these two very different diets and put them into a bar graph, the differences become more apparent.

The Zone is _Not_ a High-Protein Diet

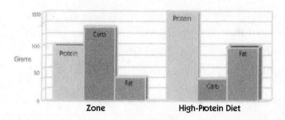

You can quickly see that no rational person could ever mistake the Zone Diet for a high-protein diet. On a high-protein diet, you are eating far more protein than carbohydrate. On the Zone, you are eating more carbohydrate than protein. On a high-protein diet, you are eating large amounts of fat, and much of that is saturated fat. On the Zone, you are eating limited amounts of fat (even though you always add some extra fat to every meal), and much of this fat is heart-healthy monounsaturated fat.

This does not mean, however, that the Zone Diet is a high-carbohydrate diet. Most high-carb diets allow you to overindulge in unfavorable carbohydrates, whereas the Zone treats these as condiments. Now that you have a basic background in hormones, let me illustrate the differences between the Zone and high-protein and high-carbohydrate diets.

High-Carbohydrate Diets

Dietary mantra: "Eat all the carbohydrates you want, just don't eat any fat."

Hormonal effect: Increased insulin levels

Consequences: Increased fat accumulation; mood swings; loss of strength; carbohydrate cravings; constant hunger; decreased mental focus; increased likelihood of heart disease, Type 2 diabetes, and cancer; and acceleration of the aging process

High-Protein Diets

Dietary mantra: "Eat all the protein you want, just don't eat any carbohydrates."

Hormonal effect: Increased glucagon levels

Consequences: Ketosis, low blood sugar, irritability, adaptation of fat cells to become "fat magnets," increased oxidation of lipids, loss of muscle mass, increased likelihood of heart disease if continued for any significant period of time, and acceleration of the aging process

The Zone

Dietary mantra: "Balance and moderation."

Hormonal effect: Keeps insulin within a zone by balancing insulin and glucagon

Consequences: Loss of excess body fat; improved control of blood sugar; increased mental and physical energy; stable moods; decreased likelihood of heart disease, Type 2 diabetes, and cancer; and slowing of the aging process

15

SCIENTIFIC VALIDATION OF THE ZONE

The Zone Diet remains one of the most misunderstood concepts in nutrition, although the concept is simple. The Zone is based on keeping various hormones generated by the macronutrient (protein, carbohydrate, and fat) composition of each meal within specified zones: not too high, not too low.

In 1995 my first book, *The Zone*, outlined the biochemical basis of the Zone Diet. However, since the publication of my dietary program, it has been incorrectly labeled as a high-protein diet, and thus linked to those risky high-protein dietary programs that have absolutely no relationship to the Zone, as explained in Chapter 14. What the Zone Diet does represent is a protein-adequate, carbohydrate-moderate, low-fat diet to keep insulin within a zone: not too high, not too low. Furthermore, the Zone Diet is based on two principles: *balance* and *moderation.* You balance the protein, carbohydrate, and fat at each meal, and consume only a moderate amount of calories at each meal.

The Zone is simply a dietary program that recommends adequate amounts of low-fat protein and lots of vegetables and fruits, with a dash of monounsaturated fat. What could be controversial about that? Yet to hear the nutritional establishment, you might think the Zone is a fad diet that is medically unsafe and nutritionally unsound.

I believe that the controversy surrounding the Zone Diet is

based on two factors. First, it forces people to consider the hormonal consequences of a meal, and in particular, how to maintain insulin within a zone. This is a totally new concept to virtually all nutritionists. Second, the Zone Diet is based on the most recent advances in medical research, which many critics seem to be totally unaware of. Recently, a number of independent studies have been published that validate the power of the Zone to change health care in America. Here is some of the most relevant recently published research. For complete information on the studies, see the references at the end of the book.

1. **The number-one risk factor that predicts heart disease is elevated insulin.** Prospective studies conducted with individuals with no initial trace of heart disease have demonstrated that elevated insulin is a vastly more powerful predictor of heart disease than is cholesterol. In fact, elevated insulin increased the likelihood of having a heart attack by a factor of 5.5, compared to elevated "bad" cholesterol (LDL), which only increased the likelihood by 2.4 times. Another prospective study has also indicated that the only blood parameter associated with increased heart attacks is increased insulin levels. A third study, from the Harvard Medical School, has demonstrated that an elevated ratio of triglycerides-to-HDL cholesterol (an indirect marker of increased insulin levels) increases the likelihood of a heart attack by a factor of 16. Therefore, any dietary program, like the Zone, that lowers insulin will decrease the risk of heart disease.

2. **The more protein you eat, the less heart disease you have.** Recent long-term studies from Harvard Medical School indicate that when the ratio of protein-to-carbohydrate reaches the levels recommended for the Zone, there is a 26 percent decrease in heart disease risk. The group that had the lowest incidence of heart disease followed a diet that provided a protein-to-carbohydrate ratio of 0.7, squarely within the boundaries of the Zone.

3. **The more protein you eat, the fewer hip fractures you get.** In postmenopausal women, a new study has indicated that women who consumed more animal protein had a 70 percent reduction in the number of hip fractures.

4. **The most powerful drug to prevent heart attacks is neither aspirin nor any cholesterol-lowering drug, but diet.** The Lyon Diet Heart Study indicated that a 70 percent reduction in both fatal and non-fatal heart attacks could be achieved simply by consuming more omega-3 fats in the diet and more fruit. This decrease in both cardiovascular mortality and overall mortality on the Lyon Diet is far greater than what was achieved by taking aspirin or any other cholesterol-lowering drug. The Zone Diet is similar to the diet used in the Lyon Diet Heart Study, except that the Zone Diet emphasizes eating greater amounts of vegetables and fruit and increasing the consumption of omega-3 fatty acids even more than does the diet used in the Lyon Diet Heart Study.

5. **Increased dietary protein is associated with increased breast cancer survival and decreased blood pressure.** As long as you decrease the consumption of fatty red meat (which is rich in arachidonic acid), the higher your intake of protein will be, and the more likely you will be to survive breast cancer. Likewise, the higher the protein intake, the lower the blood pressure.

6. **You lose body fat faster on the Zone.** In fact, the fat loss was nearly twice as great following the Zone Diet than on a high-carbohydrate diet even though both diets contained the same number of calories and the same amount of fat. This study demonstrates conclusively that a calorie is not a calorie when it comes to fat loss.

7. **The Zone Diet can initiate significant hormonal changes in only one meal.** This research work was conducted at Harvard Medical School with overweight adolescents. The Zone meal generated a completely different hormonal profile than a standard meal even though both contained the same number of calories. Furthermore, after eating a Zone meal, the number of calories consumed at the next meal was significantly less, indicating that the Zone provides better hunger control than other macronutrient compositions containing the same number of calories.

8. **The Zone Diet can reduce excess insulin levels before any fat loss is achieved.** This answers the chicken-and-egg question: Which comes first, elevated insulin or increased body fat? It has been known for some time that insulin levels can be elevated before there is any accumulation of excess body fat. However, this study demonstrated that elevated insulin levels were lowered before any fat loss was achieved, indicating that it is excess insulin that causes the accumulation of body fat.

9. **The Zone Diet can alter your genetic code.** It has been known for more than 60 years that calorie-restricted diets improve longevity. Recently, it has been shown that calorie-restricted programs can also alter the expression of the genetic code. Because it is a calorie-restricted diet, the Zone Diet is guaranteed to reverse aging, but without hunger, deprivation, or fatigue, since blood sugar levels are properly maintained.

It remains amazing to me how the media continue to ignore the science behind the Zone Diet. Even more amazing is the fact that the Zone Diet (which promotes eating 10 to 15 servings of vegetables and fruits per day with small amounts of universally recommended servings of low-fat protein, no more than 3 to 4 ounces per meal, and using monounsaturated fat as its primary fat source) is not the most highly recommended diet in America. Whatever the reasons behind this misunderstanding of the Zone Diet, you have the power to make your own decision about what type of diet you want to follow for the rest of your life. I hope this book has convinced you that it should be the Zone Diet.

THE FUTURE OF YOUR HEALTH CARE IN AMERICA

As we enter the new millennium, America's health care system stands at a crossroads. No one can honestly believe that Americans are healthier than they were 20 years ago, because we have become the fattest people on earth. New research findings indicate beyond a shadow of a doubt that the fatter you are, the more likely you are to die a premature death.

The Zone Diet was developed to address this growing crisis. The Zone is not a diet; it represents an exceptionally powerful drug for preventing the primary chronic diseases that characterize the aging process and promote premature death. The Zone Diet is also the most important tool you have to achieve permanent fat loss.

And if you are concerned about the future, then you should also be terribly concerned about what is happening to today's children. Childhood obesity has doubled in the last 15 years, adult-onset (Type 2) diabetes is now appearing in teenagers as opposed to adults over the age of 40, the growth of childhood asthma is epidemic, and there has been exponential growth in the number of children with attention-deficit disorders. A very strong argument can be made that all of these disease outbreaks in our children are consequences of growing hormonal imbalances in their diets. Children can't cook, but their parents can. If you take the time and effort to control your child's insulin levels with the food that you prepare (or let them eat), you will be ensuring a better future for your children.

Everyone understands that a good diet is your best prescription for a healthy life, yet Americans are more confused than ever about what to eat. A good diet means balance and moderation. Neither high-protein nor high-carbohydrate diets meet that criteria. The

Zone does. Hopefully, this book has cleared up much of this confusion because ultimately any diet book must be based on common sense. Hippocrates told us some 2,500 years ago that we must treat food with the same respect with which we treat any drug. His words are still true today.

As the hope fades that managed care will save us from increasing medical expenses as our population grows older, what is the future for our health care system? It's pretty bleak, unless we make some significant changes in the way we eat. It is time for us all to start taking responsibility for our own health, rather than simply relying on doctors, drugs, and expensive medical procedures to improve and prolong our lives.

Only you can feed yourself (and your children), only you can exercise, and only you can practice stress reduction. These are the components of the Anti-Aging Zone Lifestyle Pyramid. The better you put into practice these lifestyle components, the sooner you will experience a longer and better life. And the most important component of the Anti-Aging Zone Lifestyle Pyramid is eating in the Zone.

The Zone Diet is based on balance and moderation, science, and common sense. It is a simple tool, but a powerful one that can help all of us enter the millennium with healthier bodies, improved performance, and an optimistic outlook toward the future. Enter the Zone, and today can be the first day of a longer, healthier, and happier life.

RESOURCES

After reading this book, you now realize that eating in the Zone may be your most powerful "drug" for increasing daily performance (both mental and physical), losing excess body fat, and living a longer and healthier life. Although I use the term *Zone Diet*, this is not a short-term program as much as a lifelong food management system for better health through enhanced hormonal control, using foods you like to eat.

This is the sixth book I have written about the Zone technology. My first book, *The Zone*, was written primarily for cardiovascular physicians to alert them to the power of food to alter hormone levels, specifically how the levels of the hormones insulin, glucagon, and eicosanoids vary with the macronutrient composition of each meal. However, *The Zone* is not the best introduction for a beginner to understand how simple the Zone technology is to follow. That's why I usually recommend reading *Zone-Perfect Meals in Minutes* as a great introduction to Zone basics, plus *Mastering the Zone* as a more detailed how-to book for using the Zone. Once you understand basic Zone logic, then refer back to *The Zone* to better understand the biochemistry behind it. And if you really want to learn how to reverse aging and extend your life, then I strongly recommend reading *The Anti-Aging Zone*. This is my manifesto for the entire Zone technology I've developed. Although *The Anti-Aging Zone* is more complex than *The Zone*, it provides the information and motivation to make the Zone your lifelong ally to increase and enhance your longevity by reversing the aging process.

Although each of my books represents the latest research on the complex relationship between diet and hormonal response, the field is constantly changing. Much of that information can be found on my Web site, www.drsears.com, which reviews the latest updates to this rapidly evolving field. The goal of my Web site is to serve as a clearinghouse of information not only about the Zone Diet but also about worldwide hormonal research, how diet can affect various hormones, and the impact of those hormones on your longevity. Since this information is rapidly changing, I urge you to visit drsears.com to let me help you sort this new information into a digestible form (no pun intended). In addition, I am constantly updating this site with new recipes (many of them vegetarian), new research information, and simple tips to make the Zone Diet incredibly easy to follow on a lifelong basis.

Please consider drsears.com as your personal cyberspace resource to understand and easily integrate the lifestyle steps necessary to enjoy a longer and better life. If you would like additional information to show you how simple and easy Zone living can be, you can also call toll-free at 1-800-404-8171 for a free information package.

ZONE FOOD CHOICES

THE 1–2–3 METHOD

Preparing Zone meals requires an understanding of the appropriate food choices you must make for the optimal hormonal benefits. There is nothing forbidden to eat in the Zone, just as long as you maintain the right balance of protein and carbohydrate from meal to meal. However, some choices will be far better than others for maximum insulin stabilization.

If you are using the "1–2–3" method to make Zone meals, then all you have to do is balance the number of grams of fat, protein, and carbohydrate at each meal. For the typical female, this means eating about 10 grams of fat, 20 grams of protein, and 30 grams of carbohydrate at each meal. For the typical male, this means consuming about 15 grams of fat, 30 grams of protein, and 45 grams of carbohydrate at each meal. **These numbers are not set in concrete.** You may have to do some adjusting for your personal biochemistry, but they will give you a good starting point.

START WITH PROTEIN

I can't emphasize enough that every meal and snack must have adequate protein, because that will determine the amount of carbohydrate you can have without causing an overproduction of insulin. Listed below are the amounts of various protein portions that contain 10 grams of protein. The average female will need two 10-gram portions (20 grams of protein) at every meal, and the average male will need three 10-gram portions (30 grams of protein) at every meal.

Low-Fat Protein Sources

Meat and Poultry

Beef (range-fed or game)	1½ oz
Canadian bacon, lean	1½ oz
Chicken breast, skinless	1½ oz
Chicken breast, deli	2 oz
Turkey breast, skinless	1½ oz
Turkey breast, deli	2 oz
Turkey, ground	2 oz
Turkey bacon	4 strips

Fish and Seafood

Bass (freshwater)	1½ oz
Bass (sea)	2 oz
Calamari	2 oz
Catfish	2 oz
Cod	2 oz
Clams	2 oz
Crabmeat	2 oz
Haddock	2 oz
Lobster	2 oz
Mackerel	2 oz
Salmon	2 oz
Sardines	1½ oz
Scallops	2 oz
Snapper	2 oz
Trout	2 oz
Tuna (steak)	1½ oz
Tuna, canned in water	1½ oz

Eggs and Dairy

Egg whites	3 eggs
Eggs	1 egg
Egg substitutes	⅓ cup
Cottage cheese, low-fat	⅓ cup
Low-fat cheese	1½ oz
Nonfat cheese	1½ oz

Vegetarian

Protein powder	10 grams
Soybean hamburger crumbles	½ cup
Soybean Canadian bacon	5 slices
Soybean frozen sausage	1½ links
Soybean hamburger	⅔ patty
Soybean hot dog	1½ links
Tofu, extra-firm	3 oz
Tofu, firm	4 oz
Tofu, soft	6 oz

CARBOHYDRATES

Once your protein portion is set for a meal, you must balance it with carbohydrate. Each portion size listed below contains 10 grams of carbohydrate. Bear in mind that there are both favorable and unfavorable carbohydrates. The favorable carbohydrates will have the least impact on insulin secretion, whereas unfavorable carbohydrates will have a significantly higher impact even though they contain the same number of carbohydrate grams. Therefore, keep your use of unfavorable carbohydrates to a minimum.

The typical female will need three 10-gram portions of carbohydrate at each meal, whereas the typical male will need about four 10-gram portions of carbohydrate at each meal. Mix and match the carbohydrates if you wish, as long as you consume the appropriate number of 10-gram portions.

Favorable Carbohydrates (Use Primarily)

Cooked vegetables

Artichoke	4 large
Artichoke hearts	1 cup
Asparagus	12 spears
Beans, green or wax	1½ cups
Beans, black	¼ cup
Bok choy	3 cups
Broccoli	3 cups
Brussels sprouts	1½ cups

Cabbage (red or green)	3 cups
Cauliflower	4 cups
Chickpeas	¼ cup
Collard greens, chopped	2 cups
Eggplant	1½ cups
Kale	2 cups
Kidney beans	¼ cup
Leeks	1 cup
Lentils	¼ cup
Mushrooms, whole, boiled	2 cups
Onions (all types), chopped, boiled	½ cup
Okra, sliced	1 cup
Sauerkraut	1 cup
Squash, yellow, sliced, boiled	2 cups
Spinach	3½ cups
Swiss chard	2½ cups
Tomato, canned, chopped	1 cup
Tomato, pureed	½ cup
Tomato sauce	½ cup
Turnip, mashed	1½ cups
Turnip greens, chopped, boiled	4 cups
Zucchini	2 cups

Raw vegetables

Alfalfa sprouts	10 cups
Bamboo shoots	4 cups
Bean sprouts	3 cups
Beans, green	2 cups
Bell peppers (green or red)	2
Broccoli	4 cups
Brussels sprouts	1½ cups
Cabbage, shredded	4 cups
Cauliflower	4 cups
Celery, sliced	2 cups
Chickpeas	¼ cup
Cucumber (medium)	1½
Endive, chopped	10 cups
Escarole, chopped	10 cups

Jalapeño peppers	2 cups
Lettuce, iceberg	2 heads
Lettuce, romaine, shredded	10 cups
Mushrooms, chopped	4 cups
Onions, chopped	1½ cups
Radishes, sliced	4 cups
Scallions	3 cups
Shallots, diced	1½ cups
Snow peas	1½ cups
Spinach, chopped	20 cups
Tomato	2
Tomato, cherry	2 cups
Tomato, chopped	1½ cups
Water chestnuts	⅓ cup
Watercress	10 cups

Fruits (fresh, frozen, or canned light)

Apple	½
Applesauce (unsweetened)	½ cup
Apricots	3
Blackberries	¾ cup
Blueberries	½ cup
Boysenberries	½ cup
Cherries	8
Fruit cocktail, canned in water	⅓ cup
Grapes	½ cup
Grapefruit	½
Kiwi	1
Nectarine	½
Orange	½
Orange, mandarin, canned in water	⅓ cup
Peach	1
Peaches, canned in water	½ cup
Pear	½
Pineapple, cubed	½ cup
Plum	1
Raspberries	1 cup
Strawberries, diced fine	1 cup

Grains

Barley, dry	½ tablespoon
Oatmeal, slow-cooking (dry)	½ oz
Oatmeal, slow-cooking (cooked)	⅓ cup

Unfavorable Carbohydrates
(Use in Moderation)

Cooked vegetables

Acorn squash	½ cup
Beans, baked	¼ cup
Beans, refried	¼ cup
Beets, sliced	½ cup
Butternut squash	½ cup
Carrots, sliced	1 cup
Corn	¼ cup
French fries	5 pieces
Lima beans	¼ cup
Parsnips	⅓ cup
Peas	½ cup
Pinto beans	¼ cup
Potato, baked	¼
Potato, boiled	⅓ cup
Potato, mashed	¼ cup
Sweet potato, baked	⅓ cup

Fruits

Banana	⅓
Cantaloupe	¼ melon
Cranberries	¾ cup
Cranberry sauce	3 teaspoons
Dates	2 pieces
Guava	½ cup
Honeydew melon, cubed	⅔ cup
Kumquat	3 pieces
Mango, sliced	⅓ cup
Papaya, cubed	¾ cup
Pineapple, diced	½ cup

Prunes, dried	2
Raisins	1 tablespoon
Watermelon, diced	¾ cup

Fruit juices

Apple juice	⅓ cup
Apple cider	⅓ cup
Cranberry juice	¼ cup
Fruit punch	¼ cup
Grape juice	¼ cup
Grapefruit juice	⅓ cup
Lemon juice	⅓ cup
Lemonade, unsweetened	⅓ cup
Lime juice	⅓ cup
Orange juice	⅓ cup
Pineapple juice	¼ cup
Tomato juice	1 cup
Vegetable juice	¾ cup

Grains and breads

Bagel (small)	¼
Biscuit	½
Bread crumbs	½ oz
Bread, whole-grain	½ slice
Bread, white	½ slice
Breadstick, hard	1 small
Breadstick, soft	½ piece
Buckwheat, dry	½ oz
Bulgar wheat, dry	½ oz
Cereal, breakfast	½ oz
Corn bread	1 square inch piece
Cornstarch	4 teaspoons
Couscous, dry	½ oz
Cracker, graham	1½
Cracker, saltine	4
Cracker, Triscuit	3
Croissant, plain	¼
Crouton	½ oz

Donut, plain	⅓
English muffin	¼
Granola	½ oz
Grits, cooked	⅓ cup
Melba toast	½ oz
Millet, dry	½ oz
Muffin, blueberry (mini)	½
Noodles, egg (cooked)	¼ cup
Pancake (4")	1
Pasta, cooked	¼ cup
Pita bread	¼ pocket
Pita bread (mini)	½ pocket
Popcorn, popped	2 cups
Rice, brown (cooked)	⅕ cup
Rice, long-grain (cooked)	⅓ cup
Rice, white (cooked)	⅕ cup
Rice cake	1
Roll, bulky	¼
Roll, dinner (small)	½
Roll, hamburger	½
Taco shell	1
Tortilla corn (6")	1
Tortilla, flour (8")	½
Waffle	½

Others

Sugar, brown	2 teaspoons
Sugar, granulated	2 teaspoons
Sugar, confectionery	1 tablespoon
Syrup, maple	2 teaspoons
Syrup, pancake	2 teaspoons
Teriyaki sauce	1 tablespoon
Tortilla chips	½ oz

Alcohol

Beer, light	6 oz
Beer, regular	4 oz

| Distilled spirits | 1 oz |
| Wine (red or white) | 4 oz |

Add Some Fat

Now that you have balanced your protein and carbohydrate, you must add some fat. Each of the portions listed below contains 5 grams of fat. The typical female will need to add two 5-gram portions of fat to each meal, while the typical male will need to add approximately three 5-gram portions to each meal.

Best Fats (Rich in Monounsaturated Fats)

Almonds	6
Almond oil	⅔ teaspoon
Avocado	2 tablespoons
Canola oil	⅔ teaspoon
Cashews	6
Guacamole	2 tablespoons
Macadamia nuts	2
Olives, black (medium)	12
Olive oil	⅔ teaspoon
Peanuts	12
Peanut oil	⅔ teaspoon
Peanut butter, natural	1 teaspoon
Pistachios	6
Sesame oil	⅔ teaspoon
Tahini	1 tablespoon

Preparing a Zone meal is now like going to a Chinese restaurant. You choose the appropriate number of protein grams from column A (protein), balance with the appropriate number of carbohydrate portions from column B (carbohydrate), and add the appropriate number of fat grams from column C (fat). If you make your meals like this for a couple of days, you will realize that the eye-and-palm method of balancing your plate provides virtually the same results.

ZONE FOOD CHOICES

THE ZONE FOOD BLOCK METHOD

Just as with the "1–2–3" approach to making Zone meals, you can use the Zone Food Block method. Now all you have to do is add up the number of Zone blocks (instead of grams) of fat, protein, and carbohydrate at meals and then stop. For the typical female, this means eating about three Zone blocks of protein, three Zone blocks of carbohydrate, and three Zone blocks of fat at every meal. For the typical male this means consuming about four Zone blocks each of protein, carbohydrate, and fat at each meal. Again, let me emphasize that these numbers are not set in concrete. You may have to do some adjusting for your personal biochemistry, but they will give you a good starting point.

START WITH PROTEIN

I can't emphasize enough that every meal and snack has to have adequate protein, because this will determine the amount of carbohydrate Zone blocks you can have without causing an overproduction of insulin. Listed below are the sizes of various types of protein that contain one Zone block of protein, which is equivalent to 7 grams of protein. Notice this is a slightly different amount than used in the "1–2–3" method.

Low-fat Protein Sources

Meat and Poultry

Beef (range-fed or game)	1 oz
Canadian bacon, lean	1 oz
Chicken breast, skinless	1 oz

Chicken breast, deli	1½ oz
Turkey breast, skinless	1 oz
Turkey breast, deli	1½ oz
Turkey, ground	1½ oz
Turkey bacon	3 strips

Fish and Seafood

Bass (freshwater)	1 oz
Bass (sea)	1½ oz
Calamari	1½ oz
Catfish	1½ oz
Cod	1½ oz
Clams	1½ oz
Crabmeat	1½ oz
Haddock	1½ oz
Lobster	1½ oz
Mackerel	1½ oz
Salmon	1½ oz
Sardines	1 oz
Scallops	1½ oz
Snapper	1½ oz
Trout	1½ oz
Tuna (steak)	1 oz
Tuna, canned in water	1 oz

Eggs and Dairy

Egg whites	2 eggs
Eggs	1 egg
Egg substitutes	¼ cup
Cottage cheese, low-fat	¼ cup
Low-fat cheese	1 oz
Nonfat cheese	1 oz

Vegetarian

Protein powder	7 grams
Soybean hamburger crumbles	⅓ cup
Soybean Canadian bacon	3 slices
Soybean frozen sausage	1 link

Soybean hamburger	½ patty
Soybean hot dog	1 link
Tofu, extra-firm	2 oz
Tofu, firm	3 oz
Tofu, soft	4 oz

CARBOHYDRATES

Once you have determined the number of Zone blocks of protein you plan to consume for a meal, you have to balance it with carbohydrate. Each Zone block of carbohydrate contains 9 grams of carbohydrate. Notice this is slightly different than the "1–2–3" method. Bear in mind that there are both favorable and unfavorable carbohydrates. The favorable carbohydrates will have the least impact on insulin secretion, whereas unfavorable carbohydrates will have a significantly higher impact even though they contain the same number of grams of carbohydrate. Thus, keep your use of unfavorable carbohydrates to a minimum.

The typical female will need three Zone blocks of carbohydrate at each meal, whereas the typical male will need four Zone blocks of carbohydrate at each meal. The following portion sizes represent one Zone block of carbohydrate.

FAVORABLE CARBOHYDRATES
(USE PRIMARILY)

Cooked Vegetables

Artichoke	4 large
Artichoke hearts	1 cup
Asparagus	12 spears
Beans, green or wax	1½ cups
Beans, black	¼ cup
Bok choy	3 cups
Broccoli	3 cups
Brussels sprouts	1½ cups
Cabbage (red or green)	3 cups
Cauliflower	4 cups
Chickpeas	¼ cup

Collard greens, chopped	2 cups
Eggplant	1½ cups
Kale	2 cups
Kidney beans	¼ cup
Leeks	1 cup
Lentils	¼ cup
Mushrooms, whole, boiled	2 cups
Onions (all types), chopped, boiled	½ cup
Okra, sliced	1 cup
Sauerkraut	1 cup
Squash, yellow, sliced, boiled	2 cups
Spinach	3½ cups
Swiss chard	2½ cups
Tomato, canned, chopped	1 cup
Tomato, pureed	½ cup
Tomato sauce	½ cup
Turnip, mashed	1½ cups
Turnip greens, chopped, boiled	4 cups
Zucchini	2 cups

Raw Vegetables

Alfalfa sprouts	10 cups
Bamboo shoots	4 cups
Bean sprouts	3 cups
Beans, green	2 cups
Bell peppers (green or red)	2
Broccoli	4 cups
Brussels sprouts	1½ cups
Cabbage, shredded	4 cups
Cauliflower	4 cups
Celery, sliced	2 cups
Chickpeas	¼ cup
Cucumber (medium)	1½
Endive, chopped	10 cups
Escarole, chopped	10 cups
Jalapeño peppers	2 cups
Lettuce, iceberg	2 heads
Lettuce, romaine, shredded	10 cups

Mushrooms, chopped	4 cups
Onions, chopped	1½ cups
Radishes, sliced	4 cups
Scallions	3 cups
Shallots, diced	1½ cups
Snow peas	1½ cups
Spinach, chopped	20 cups
Tomato	2
Tomato, cherry	2 cups
Tomato, chopped	1½ cups
Water chestnuts	⅓ cup
Watercress	10 cups

Fruits (fresh, frozen, or canned light)

Apple	½
Applesauce (unsweetened)	⅓ cup
Apricots	3
Blackberries	¾ cup
Blueberries	½ cup
Boysenberries	½ cup
Cherries	8
Fruit cocktail, canned in water	⅓ cup
Grapes	½ cup
Grapefruit	½
Kiwi	1
Nectarine	½
Orange	½
Orange, mandarin, canned in water	⅓ cup
Peach	1
Peaches, canned in water	½ cup
Pear	½
Pineapple, cubed	½ cup
Plum	1
Raspberries	1 cup
Strawberries, diced fine	1 cup

Grains

| Barley, dry | ½ tablespoon |

Oatmeal, slow-cooking (dry)   ½ oz
Oatmeal, slow-cooking (cooked)   ⅓ cup

UNFAVORABLE CARBOHYDRATES (USE IN MODERATION)

Cooked Vegetables

Acorn squash	½ cup
Beans, baked	¼ cup
Beans, refried	¼ cup
Beets, sliced	½ cup
Butternut squash	½ cup
Carrots, sliced	1 cup
Corn	¼ cup
French fries	5 pieces
Lima beans	¼ cup
Parsnips	⅓ cup
Peas	½ cup
Pinto beans	¼ cup
Potato, baked	¼
Potato, boiled	⅓ cup
Potato, mashed	¼ cup
Sweet potato, baked	⅓ cup

Fruits

Banana	⅓
Cantaloupe	¼ melon
Cranberries	¾ cup
Cranberry sauce	3 teaspoons
Dates	2 pieces
Guava	½ cup
Honeydew melon, cubed	⅔ cup
Kumquat	3 pieces
Mango, sliced	⅓ cup
Papaya, cubed	¾ cup
Pineapple, diced	½ cup
Prunes, dried	2

Raisins	1 tablespoon
Watermelon, diced	¾ cup

Fruit Juices

Apple juice	⅓ cup
Apple cider	⅓ cup
Cranberry juice	¼ cup
Fruit punch	¼ cup
Grape juice	¼ cup
Grapefruit juice	⅓ cup
Lemon juice	⅓ cup
Lemonade, unsweetened	⅓ cup
Lime juice	⅓ cup
Orange juice	⅓ cup
Pineapple juice	¼ cup
Tomato juice	1 cup
Vegetable juice	¾ cup

Grains and Breads

Bagel (small)	¼
Biscuit	½
Bread crumbs	½ oz
Bread, whole-grain	½ slice
Bread, white	½ slice
Bread stick, hard	1 small
Bread stick, soft	½ piece
Buckwheat, dry	½ oz
Bulgar wheat, dry	½ oz
Cereal, breakfast	½ oz
Corn Bread	1 square inch piece
Cornstarch	4 teaspoons
Couscous, dry	½ oz
Cracker, graham	1½
Cracker, saltine	4
Cracker, Triscuit	3
Croissant, plain	¼
Crouton	½ oz
Donut, plain	⅓

English muffin	¼
Granola	½ oz
Grits, cooked	⅓ cup
Melba toast	½ oz
Millet, dry	½ oz
Muffin, blueberry (mini)	½
Noodles, egg (cooked)	¼ cup
Pancake (4")	1
Pasta, cooked	¼ cup
Pita bread	¼ pocket
Pita bread, mini	½ pocket
Popcorn, popped	2 cups
Rice, brown (cooked)	⅕ cup
Rice, long-grain (cooked)	⅓ cup
Rice, white (cooked)	⅕ cup
Rice cake	1
Roll, bulky	¼
Roll, dinner (small)	½
Roll, hamburger	½
Taco shell	1
Tortilla, corn (6")	1
Tortilla, flour (8")	½
Waffle	½

Others

Barbecue sauce	2 tablespoons
Cake (small slice)	⅓
Candy bar (regular)	¼
Catsup	2 tablespoons
Cocktail sauce	2 tablespoons
Cookie (small)	1
Honey	½ tablespoon
Ice cream, regular	¼ cup
Ice cream, premium	⅕ cup
Jam or jelly	2 tablespoons
Plum sauce	1½ tablespoons
Molasses, light	½ tablespoon
Potato chips	½ oz

Pretzels	½ oz
Relish, pickle	4 teaspoons
Salsa	½ cup
Sugar, brown	2 teaspoons
Sugar, granulated	2 teaspoons
Sugar, confectionery	1 tablespoon
Syrup, maple	2 teaspoons
Syrup, pancake	2 teaspoons
Teriyaki sauce	1 tablespoon
Tortilla chips	½ oz

Alcohol

Beer, light	6 oz
Beer, regular	4 oz
Distilled spirits	1 oz
Wine (red or white)	4 oz

Add Some Fat

Now that you have balanced your protein and carbohydrate Zone blocks, you have to add some fat. Each of these portion sizes of fat contains 3 grams of fat, which is again different from the "1–2–3" method. The typical female will need to add three Zone blocks of fat to each meal, whereas the typical male will need to add approximately four Zone blocks of fat to each meal.

Best Fats (Rich in Monounsaturated Fats)

Almonds	3
Almond oil	⅓ teaspoon
Avocado	1 tablespoon
Canola oil	⅓ teaspoon
Cashews	3
Guacamole	1 tablespoon
Macadamia nuts	1
Olives, black (medium)	4
Olive oil	⅓ teaspoon
Peanuts	6
Peanut oil	⅓ teaspoon

Peanut butter, natural	½ tablespoon
Pistachios	3
Sesame oil	⅓ teaspoon
Tahini	½ tablespoon

Preparing a Zone meal is once again like going to a Chinese restaurant. You choose the appropriate number of Zone blocks from column A (protein), balance with the appropriate number of Zone blocks from column B (carbohydrate), and add the appropriate number of Zone blocks from column C (fat). As with the "1–2–3" method, if you make your meals like this for a couple of days, you will realize that the eye-and-palm method of balancing your plate provides virtually the same results.

BIBLIOGRAPHY

Chapter 1: What Is the Zone?

"Guidelines call more Americans overweight." *Harvard Health Letter* 10:7 (1998).

"New guidelines mean more Americans are overweight." *Mayo Clinic Health Letter* 9:4 (1998).

Sears, B. *The Zone*. New York: ReganBooks, 1995.

Chapter 2: Food and Hormones

Bruning, P.F., J.M.G. Bonfrer, P.A.H. van Noord, A.A.M. Hart, M. de Jong-Bakker, and W.J. Nooijen. "Insulin resistance and breast cancer." *International Journal of Cancer* 52:511–516 (1992).

Depres, J.-P., B. Lamarche, P. Mauriege, B. Cantin, G.R. Dagenais, K.S. Moorjani, and P.J. Lupien. "Hyperinsulinemia as an independent risk factor for ischemic heart disease." *New England Journal of Medicine* 334:952–957 (1996).

Gaziano, J.M., C.H. Hennekens, C.H. O'Donnell, J.L. Breslow, and J.E. Buring. "Fasting triglycerides, high-density lipoproteins, and risk of myocardial infarction." *Circulation* 96:2520–2525 (1997).

Heini, A.F. and R.L. Weinsier. "Divergent trends in obesity and fat intake patterns: An American paradox." *American Journal of Medicine* 102:259–264 (1997).

Hollenbeck, C. and G.M. Reaven. "Variations in insulin stimulated glucose uptake in healthy individuals with normal glucose tolerance." *Journal of Clinical Endocrinology and Metabolism* 64:1169–1173 (1987).

Holmes, M.D., M.J. Stampfer, G.A. Colditz, B. Rosner, D.J. Hunter, and W.C. Willett. "Dietary factors and the survival of women with breast cancer." *Cancer* 86:751–753 (1999).

Lamarch, B., A. Tchernot, P. Mauriege, B. Cantin, P.-J. Lupien, and J.-P. Depres. "Fasting insulin and apolipoprotein B levels and low density particle size as risk factors for ischemic heart disease." *Journal of the American Medical Association* 279: 1955–1961 (1998).

Markovic, T.P., A.B. Jenkins, L.V. Campbell, S.M. Furler, E.W. Kragen, and D.J. Chisholm. "The determinants of glycemic responses to diet restriction and weight loss in obesity and NIDDM." *Diabetes Care* 21:687–694 (1998).

Munger, R.G., J.R. Cerhan, and B.C.-H. Chiu. "Prospective study of dietary protein intake and risk of hip fracture in postmenopausal women." *American Journal of Clinical Nutrition* 69:147–152 (1999).

Pelikonova, T., M. Kohout, J. Base, Z. Stefka, J. Kovar, L. Kerdova, and J. Valek. "Effect of acute hyperinsulinemia on fatty acid composition of serum lipids in non-insulin dependent diabetics and healthy men." *Clinica Chimica Acta* 203:329–337 (1991).

Schapira, D.V., N.B. Kumar, G.H. Lyman, and C.E. Cox. "Abdominal obesity and breast cancer risk." *Annals of Internal Medicine* 112:182–186 (1990).

Sears, B. *The Zone*. New York: ReganBooks, 1995.

Sears, B. *Mastering the Zone*. New York: ReganBooks, 1997.

Sears, B. *Zone-Perfect Meals in Minutes*. New York: ReganBooks, 1997.

Sears, B. *The Anti-Aging Zone*. New York: ReganBooks, 1999.

Stoll, B.A. "Western nutrition and the insulin resistance syndrome: a link to breast cancer." *European Journal of Clinical Nutrition* 53:83–87 (1999).

Stoll, B.A. "Essential fatty acids, insulin resistance, and breast cancer risk." *Nutr Cancer* 31:72–77 (1998).

Chapter 3: Getting Started in the Zone

Ascherio, A., C.H. Hennekens, J.E. Buring, C. Master, M.J. Stampfer, and W.C. Willett. "Trans-fatty acids intake and risk of myocardial infarction." *Circulation* 89:94–101 (1994).

Ascherio, A. and W.C. Willett. "Health effects of trans-fatty acids." *American Journal of Clinical Nutrition* 66:1006S–1010S (1997).

Ascherio, A., M.B. Katan, P.L. Zock, M.J. Stampfer, and W.C. Willett. "Trans-fatty acids and coronary heart disease." *New England Journal of Medicine* 340:1994–1998 (1999).

Sears, B. *The Zone*. New York: ReganBooks, 1995.

Sears, B. *Mastering the Zone*. New York: ReganBooks, 1997.

Sears, B. *Zone-Perfect Meals in Minutes*. New York: ReganBooks, 1997.

Sears, B. *The Anti-Aging Zone*. New York: ReganBooks, 1999.

Sears, B. *The Soy Zone*. New York: ReganBooks, 2000.

Silver, M.J., W. Hoch, J.J. Koesis, C.M. Ingerman, and J.B. Smith. "Arachidonic acid causes sudden death in rabbits." *Science* 183:1035–1037 (1974).

Chapter 4: A Zone Makeover for Your Kitchen

Sears, B. *Zone-Perfect Meals in Minutes*. New York: ReganBooks, 1997.

Chapter 8: The Soy Zone

Kagawa, Y. "Impact of Westernization on the nutrition of Japanese: Changes in physique, cancer, longevity, and centenarians." *Preventive Medicine* 7:205–217 (1978).

Mimura, G., K. Murakami, and M. Gushiken. "Nutritional factors for longevity in Okinawa—present and future." *Nutritional Health* 8:159–163 (1992).

Sears, B. *The Soy Zone*. New York: ReganBooks, 2000.

Weindruch, R. and R.L. Walford. *The Retardation of Aging and Disease by Dietary Restriction*. Springfield, IL: Charles C. Thomas, 1988.

Weindruch, R. "Caloric restriction and aging." *Scientific American* 274: 46–52 (1996).

Chapter 9: The Anti-Aging Zone

Sears, B. *The Anti-Aging Zone*. New York: ReganBooks, 1999.

Chapter 10: Zone Supplements

Sears, B. *Zone-Perfect Meals in Minutes*. New York: ReganBooks, 1997.

Chapter 11: Fine-Tuning the Zone

Sears, B. *Mastering the Zone*. New York: ReganBooks, 1997.

Chapter 13: Frequently Asked Questions

American Heart Association. *Heart and Stroke Facts*. 1997 Statistical Supplement. American Heart Association, Dallas, TX (1998).

Kekwick, A. and G.L.S. Pawan. "Calorie intake in relation to body-weight changes in the obese." *Lancet* ii:155–161 (1956).

Holt, S., J. Brand, C. Soveny, and J. Hansky. "Relationship of satiety to postprandial glycemic, insulin, and cholecystokinin responses." *Appetite* 18:129–141 (1992).

Hunt, J.R., S.K. Gallagher, L.K. Johnson, and G.I. Lykken. "High- versus low-meat diets: effects on zinc absorption, iron status, and calcium, copper, iron, magnesium, manganese, nitrogen, phosphorous, and zinc balance in postmenopausal women." *American Journal of Clinical Nutrition* 62:621–632 (1995).

Mallick, N.P. "Dietary protein and progression of chronic renal disease: Large randomized controlled trial suggest no benefit from restriction." *British Medical Journal* 309:1101–1102 (1994).

Munger, R.G., J.R. Cerhan, and B. Chiu. "Prospective study of dietary protein and risk of hip fracture in postmenopausal women." *American Journal of Clinical Nutrition* 69:147–152 (1999).

Phinney, S.D., P.G. Davis, S.B. Johnson, and R.T. Holman. "Obesity and weight loss alter polyunsaturated metabolism in humans." *American Journal of Clinical Nutrition* 52:831–838 (1991).

Renauld, S. and M. de Lorgeril. "Wine, alcohol, platelets and the French paradox for coronary heart disease." *Lancet* 339:1523–1528 (1992).

Sears, B. *The Zone*. New York: ReganBooks, 1995.

Serra-Majem, L., L. Ribas, R. Tresserras, and L. Salleras. "How could changes in diet explain changes in coronary heart disease mortality in Spain? The Spanish paradox." *American Journal of Clinical Nutrition* 61: 1351S–1359S (1995).

Spencer, H., L. Kramer, M. DeBartolo, C. Morris, and D. Osis. "Further studies on the effect of a high protein diet as meat on calcium metabolism." *American Journal of Clinical Nutrition* 37:924–929 (1983).

Spencer, H., L. Kramer, and D. Osis. "Do protein and phosphorus cause calcium loss?" *Journal of Nutrition* 118:657–660 (1988).

Chapter 14: Why High-Protein Diets Fail

Folsom, A.R., J. Ma, P.G. McGovern, and H. Eckfeldt. "Relation between plasma phospholipid saturated fatty acids and hyper-insulinemia." *Metabolism* 45:223–228 (1996).

Jain, S.K., K. Kannan, and G. Lim. "Ketosis (acetoacetate) can generate oxygen radicals and cause increased lipid peroxidation and growth inhibition in human endothelial cells." *Free Radical Biology and Medicine* 25:1083–1088 (1998).

Jain, S.K., R. McVie, R. Jackson, S.N. Levine, and G. Lim. "Effect of hyperketonemia on plasma lipid peroxidation levels in diabetic patients." *Diabetes Care* 22:1171–1175 (1999).

Jain, S.K. and R. McVie. "Hyperketonemia can increase lipid peroxidation and lower glutathione levels in hu in erythrocytes in vitro and in Type 1 diabetic patients." *Di etes* 48:1850–1855 (1999).

Kern, P.A., J.M. Ong, B. Soffan, and J. Carty. "The effects of weight loss on the activity and expression of adipose-tissue lipoprotein lipase in very obese individuals." *New England Journal of Medicine* 322:1053–1059 (1990).

Storlien, L.H., A.B. Jenkins, D.J. Chisholm, W.S. Pascoe, S. Khouri, and E.W. Kraegen. "Influence of dietary fat composition on development of insulin resistance in rats. Relationship to muscle triglyceride and omega-3 fatty acids in muscle phospholipid." *Diabetes* 40:280–289 (1991).

Storlien, L.H., D.A. Pan, A.D. Kriketos, J. O'Connor, I.D. Caterson, G.J. Cooney, A.B. Jenkins, and L.A. Baur. "Skeletal muscle membrane lipids and insulin resistance." *Lipids* 31:S261–265 (1996).

Chapter 15: Scientific Validation of the Zone

Boyko E.J., D.L. Leonetti, R.W. Bergestrom, L. Newell-Morris, and W.Y. Fujimoto. "Low insulin secretion and high-fasting insulin and c-peptide predict increased visceral adiposity." *Diabetes* 45:1010–1015 (1996).

De Lorgeril, M., P. Salen, J.-L. Martin, I. Monjaud, J. Delaye, and N. Mamelle. "Mediterranean diet, traditional risk factors, and rate of cardiovascular complications after myocardial infarction. Final report of the Lyon Diet Heart Study." *Circulation* 99:779–785 (1999).

Depres, J.-P., B. Lamarche, P. Mauriege, B. Cantin, G.R. Dagenais, S. Moorjani, and P.-J. Pupien. "Hyperinsulinemia as an independent risk factor for ischemic heart disease." *New England Journal of Medicine* 334:952–957 (1996).

Gaziano, J.M., C.H. Hennekens, C.H. O'Donnell, J.L. Breslow, and J.E. Buring. "Fasting triglycerides, high-density lipoproteins, and risk of myocardial infarction." *Circulation* 96:2520–2525 (1997).

Haffner, S.M., R.A. Valdez, H.P. Hazuda, B.D. Mitchell, P.A. Morales, and M.P. Stern. "Prospective analysis of the insulin-resistance syndrome (syndrome X)." *Diabetes* 41:715–722 (1992).

Holmes, M.D., M.J. Stampfer, G.A. Colditz, B. Rosner, D.J. Hunter, and W.C. Willett. "Dietary factors and the survival of women with breast cancer." *Cancer* 86:751–753 (1999).

Hu, F.B., M.J. Stampfer, J.E. Manson, E. Rimm, G.A. Colditz, F.E. Speizer, C.H. Hennekens, and W.C. Willett. "Dietary protein and the risk of ischemic heart disease in women." *American Journal of Clinical Nutrition* 70:221–227 (1999).

Lamarch, B., A. Tchernot, P. Mauriege, B. Cantin, P.-J. Lupien, and J.-P. Depres. "Fasting insulin and apolipoprotein B levels and low density particle size as risk factors for ischemic heart disease." *Journal of the American Medical Association* 279: 1955–1961 (1998).

Lee, C.-K., R.G. Klopp, R. Weindruch, and T.A. Prolla. "Gene expression profile of aging and its retardation by caloric restriction." *Science* 285:1390–1393 (1999).

Ludwig, D.S., J.A. Majzoub, A. Al-Zahrani, G.E. Dallal, I. Blanco, and S.B. Roberts. "High glycemic index foods, overeating, and obesity." *Pediatrics* 103:E26 (1999).

Markovic, T.P., A.B. Jenkins, L.V. Campbell, S.M. Furler, E.W. Kraegen, and D.J. Chisholm. "The determinants of glycemic response to diet restriction and weight loss in obesity and NIDDM." *Diabetes Care* 21:687–694 (1998).

Munger, R.G., J.R. Cerhan, and B.C.-H. Chiu. "Prospective study of dietary protein intake and risk of hip fracture in postmenopausal women." *American Journal of Clinical Nutrition* 69:147–152 (1999).

Odeleye O.D., M. de Courten, D.J. Pettit, and E. Ravassin. "Fasting hyperinsulinemia is a predictor of increased body weight gain and obesity in Pima Indian children." *Diabetes* 46:1341–1345 (1997).

Scandinavian Simvastatin Survival Study Group. "Randomized trial of cholesterol lowering in 4,444 patients with coronary heart disease: The Scandinavian simvastatin survival study (4S)." *Lancet* 344:1383–1389 (1994).

Skov, A.R., S. Toubro, B. Ronn, L. Holm, and A. Astrup. "Randomized trial on protein vs carbohydrate in ad libitum fat reduced diet for the treatment of obesity." *International Journal of Obesity* 23:528–536 (1999).

Stamler, J., P. Elliott, H. Kesteloot, R. Nichols, G. Claeys, A.R. Dyer, and M.A. Stamler. "Inverse relation of dietary protein markers with blood pressure." *Circulation* 94:1629–1634 (1996).

Steering Committee of the Physician Health Study Research Group. "Preliminary report findings from the aspirin component of the ongoing physician health study." *New England Journal of Medicine* 320:262–264 (1988).

Zavaroni, I., E. Bonora, M. Pagliara, E. Dall'aglio, L. Luchetti, G. Buonanno, P.A. Bonati, M. Bergonzani, L. Gnudi, M. Passeri, and G. Reaven. "Risk factors for coronary artery disease in healthy persons with hyperinsulinemia and normal glucose tolerance." *New England Journal of Medicine* 320:702–706 (1989).

INDEX